the Allergy Exclusion Diet

OTHER HAY HOUSE TITLES
OF RELATED INTEREST

Books

The Body Knows: *How to Tune In to Your Body and Improve Your Health,* by Caroline Sutherland, Medical Intuitive

Eating in the Light: *Making Your Way to Vegetarianism on Your Spiritual Path,* by Doreen Virtue, Ph.D., and Becky Prelitz, M.F.T., R.D.

Healing with Herbs and Home Remedies A–Z, by Hanna Kroeger

Homeopathy A–Z, by Dana Ullman, M.P.H.

Vegetarian Meals for People-on-the-Go: *101 Quick & Easy Recipes,* by Vimala Rodgers

Wheat-Free, Worry-Free: *The Art of Happy, Healthy, Gluten-Free Living,* by Danna Korn

Audio Programs

Body Talk: *No-Nonsense, Common-Sense, Sixth-Sense Solutions to Create Health and Healing,* by Mona Lisa Schulz, M.D., Ph.D., and Christiane Northrup, M.D.

Eating Wisdom, by Andrew Weil, M.D., with Michael Toms

Your Diet, Your Health, with Christiane Northrup, M.D.

All of the above are available at your local bookstore, or may be ordered through Hay House, Inc.:

(800) 654-5126 or **(760) 431-7695**
(800) 650-5115 (fax) or **(760) 431-6948 (fax)**
www.hayhouse.com

the Allergy Exclusion Diet

**The 28-day plan
to solve your food
intolerances**

JILL CARTER AND ALISON EDWARDS

Hay House, Inc.
Carlsbad, California • Sydney, Australia
Canada • Hong Kong • United Kingdom

Published and distributed in the United States by:
Hay House, Inc., P.O. Box 5100, Carlsbad, CA 92018-5100 • (800) 654-5126 • (800) 650-5115 (fax)
www.hayhouse.com • Hay House Australia Pty Ltd, P.O. Box 515, Brighton-Le-Sands,
NSW 2216 • *phone:* 1800 023 516 • *e-mail:* info@hayhouse.com.au

Designed by: Lovelock & Co.

First published in 2002 by Vermilion, an imprint of Ebury Press, Random House,
20 Vauxhall Bridge Road, London SW1V 2SA • www.randomhouse.co.uk
• ISBN: 0 09 188221 4

Library of Congress Cataloging-in-Publication Data

Carter, Jill.
  The allergy exclusion diet : the 28-day plan to solve your food
intolerances / Jill Carter and Alison Edwards.
    p. cm.
Includes index.
  ISBN 1-40190-102-6
  1. Food allergy—Diet therapy. I. Edwards, Alison, 1928— II. Title.
  RC588.D53 C358 2003
  616.97'50654—dc21

                                2002007712

                          ISBN 1-4019-0102-6

                  06 05 04 03   4 3 2 1
                1st Hay House printing, February 2003

                Printed in the United States of America

A note to the reader

The information contained in this book is given for the purposes of helping people
who suspect they may have a food allergy or intolerance. Before following the
advice, the reader is advised to give careful consideration to the nature of their
problem and to consult a health-care practitioner if in any doubt. This is
particularly important for dealing with babies and young children, and in cases of
diabetes, severe depression, and schizophrenia. This book should not be used as a
substitute for medical treatment, and while every care has been taken to ensure
the accuracy of the information, the authors and publishers cannot accept any
responsibility for any problems arising out of experimentation
with the method described.

contents

introduction

Poised on the threshold of change, your mind whirls around those favorite foods you love and crave – the chocolates, the pizzas, the ice creams, and the snacks. Could there really be some "hidden enemy" lurking in such delicacies? Could a simple food allergy to these foods be spoiling your life? Could you reduce your dependency on painkillers, antacids, and all those other palliative medicines just by altering your diet?

The answer, quite simply, is yes. This book will first explain how food allergies can affect you, and second, will show you how to alleviate them. It will then guide you through the Elimination Diet, giving you recipes for each meal. This will enable you to discover the hidden culprits that are preventing you from feeling as well as you can.

If you are already allergic or intolerant to certain foods, you will probably become allergic to others, because if a food is eaten too frequently, the body is unable to break it down and process it completely. It can, therefore, become overloaded. Even if you don't suffer from allergies, it is likely that you

Case study

Jack, age six, was constantly bothered by weeping eczema. Twice he was admitted to hospital as a toddler, and on one occasion he had scratched himself so badly that he had to be sedated. Then his mother discovered he was intolerant to all dairy products and all legumes. Almost overnight he started to improve. For the first time since he was born, he started to sleep through the night, his yellow sores disappeared, and he became a different child.

will feel the effects of the overload. This is where the Rotation Diet, which follows the Elimination Diet, comes in.

A rotation diet offers a way of spacing foods out so you can recover from the effects of a food before it is eaten again. It was originally designed to help people who are allergic to foods, but it can be wonderfully beneficial for everyone. Many people with highly demanding lifestyles find that their energy levels increase, and they feel much better when they rotate their foods. After all, it was not so long ago that we depended on food grown close at hand, and the seasons of the year dictated a natural rotation.

If you have discovered that you are allergic to certain foods, either as a result of following the Elimination Diet, or from the many tests available, it is important that you understand how to plan and use a rotation diet. However, the prospect of embarking on a rotation diet can be so daunting that all but the most determined have either given up in the early stages or not started at all. This book will give you a clear understanding of the principles, and show you just how to follow them. Once grasped, the diet can then be adapted to your individual needs. With delicious and nourishing recipes for you to experiment with and enjoy, this book will give you the chance to sample foods that you may never have thought to try before.

There is good news for weight watchers, too. Eliminating food allergies and then following the Rotation Diet could be the critical

Daphne (eight years old) was constantly missing school due to persistent headaches, diarrhea, and tummy aches. She was referred to her local hospital, and after counseling treatment failed, she was referred to a dietitian who put her on a milk, egg, beef, and poultry-free diet. When this did not help, she was advised to stop all preservatives. Her mother then found a natural medicine center and a test revealed reactions to wheat, oats, barley, and rye. Because there had been a long history of illness a rotation diet was recommended. Milk, eggs, beef and poultry were returned to the diet in the rotation but the cereal grains were strictly avoided. Her mother wrote a report stating "no headaches and tummy aches; no time away from school; she attended willingly and happily every day and her general complexion is now pink and healthy rather than the black eyes and a white face. She has had no diarrhea for eight weeks.

move needed to lose those extra pounds or, if you are underweight, to establishing your ideal weight.

If you have been a migraine, eczema, or asthma sufferer for years; if you are experiencing pain and stiffness creeping into muscles and joints; if you have digestive problems or if you suffer from depression, mood changes, and fatigue; if you have sinus problems, earache, tinnitus, or permanent catarrh; if you are concerned because your child is overactive and unable to sleep, or if you have any of the symptoms listed in the next chapter, then this book could be the answer for you and a major step toward enhancing not only your own health but also the health of others around you.

chapter 1
an understanding
of allergies

It is useful to understand exactly what allergies are, the way they can affect you and their possible causes. The word *allergy* has become a catchword, particularly in connection with food. What we are usually talking about, though, is a food intolerance rather than an allergy.

If you were to have a "true" allergic reaction to a food, you would know about it immediately, as the initial response can be very dramatic. With this type of abnormal hypersensitivity, your body's defense mechanisms would be alerted. Hives, rashes, and puffy eyes could appear within seconds; an asthmatic attack, swelling of joints, vomiting, and nausea could then follow; and, in some severe cases, anaphylactic shock or an apparent heart attack. Classic foods that cause this type of reaction are shellfish, strawberries, cashews, and peanuts. If you are allergic to something, a reaction will occur each time the particular food is eaten. The condition is well recognized by doctors, and laboratory tests can confirm the culprits. The problem is then overcome simply by avoiding the offending food.

The words *intolerance* and *sensitivity* are both used to describe the other type of allergy, of which orthodox medicine now recognizes the existence. According to the Royal College of Physicians and the British Nutritional Foundation, "an intolerance is a reaction caused by a food, but the mechanism is not clear." It seems that an intolerance, like an allergy, may also result from a misdirected response of the body's immune system, but the reactions are less apparent. The immune system, which is designed to protect your body from invading organisms such as bacteria and viruses, makes antibodies, which kill or neutralize the invaders. In people with allergies, however, the antibodies attack normally harmless substances such as food. This is when a reaction occurs. As you continue to eat the substance, though, perhaps even two or three times a day, your body will endeavor to adapt. Your reactions will become reduced and the symptoms masked, therefore presenting a far more vague and complex picture, so much so that you may have difficulty associating these symptoms with the foods you are eating.

You will often crave and become addicted to the particular food to which you are intolerant. You can give up anything else, you may say, but not my morning cup of coffee, glass of wine, or buttered toast. You may not consciously realize your craving, but will be regularly filling yourself up with the particular food to satisfy your yearnings. This is because you will usually experience a "lift" after eating a food to which you are intolerant, as your body will be producing large amounts of adrenaline to fight the reaction. However, the beneficial feeling will then disappear after one or two hours. As time goes by, and your body starts to get tired from so much overstimulation, you will need more and more of the food to feel good. In extreme cases, this process is similar to drug, alcohol, and cigarette addiction.

If you continue to subject your body to the food for long enough, you can reach a stage of exhaustion. Collapsing over your desk at work, suffering "burnout" before your years, or simply cutting short your shopping trip—these are all signs that your body's defense mechanism can no longer cope.

The causes of allergies and food intolerances

Allergies and food intolerances are on the increase. This may be due to a number of factors, of which pollution is one. Today, we are exposed to more chemicals than ever before: in the air we breathe; in the chemically contaminated food, water, and prescription medicines we ingest; and from the many toxic substances that our skin comes into contact with. Our daily diet contains pesticides, mycotoxins, dyes, additives, and many other chemicals. In addition, heavy metals such as lead from gas fumes and mercury from amalgam tooth fillings can overload the natural detoxifying pathways of the body, particularly in the liver. The result is that the defense systems of the body become overworked and overextended, and so, not surprisingly, fail to work efficiently.

Nutritional deficiency can also play a part. The increasing use of chemicals in farming, as well as the transport, processing, and storage of foods for long periods can all lead to the decrease of valuable vitamins and minerals in foods. These vitamins and minerals are vital for a strong immune system, and since there is a noticeable correlation between immune deficiency and allergies, it is probable that if you have allergies or intolerances, you will be deficient in many vitamins and minerals. This is particularly likely if you eat a lot of refined sugar, milk, and wheat, since these foods can deplete your vitamin and mineral levels. Approximately 48 percent of the raw molasses extracted from sugar cane consists of vitamins and minerals that are necessary for the body to break down and metabolize the sugar molecules. However, most people eat white processed sugar, which has none of these nutrients left, so eating this will actually draw on the body's reserves of minerals and vitamins. Wheat, which is high in gluten, a sticky, gluey-like substance, can coat the lining of the intestines and therefore prevent the proper absorption of nutrients from the diet. Similarly, milk can damage the lining of the intestines.

Sugar and wheat can also encourage an overgrowth of unfriendly microorganisms such as candida albicans in the gut. Candida is a yeast growth present in and on most people. It is normally controlled by the immune defenses and the "friendly flora" in the intestines. When the immune system has been weakened, for example by a chronic viral infection such as glandular fever, or the internal flora has been depleted, perhaps by antibiotics or contraceptive pills, the candida can grow out of control and the condition called candidiasis manifests. This condition affects the mucous membranes and allows undigested food particles to pass through the walls of the intestines and trigger food intolerances. Parasites such as giardia lamblia may also trigger food intolerances in the same way by damaging the intestines and destroying the friendly bacteria.

Another contributory factor to allergies and food intolerances may be bottle-feeding with cow's milk. An infant's intestinal tract is very porous, and it takes between six to twelve months before it can screen out the large molecules in substances such as wheat, milk products, fish, and egg whites. So, if a baby is fed on cow's milk or solid food during the early months, its digestive system may not be able to cope. In addition, it will be missing the protective substances in the mother's milk and colostrum, so it will not be able to build up a healthy immune system.

There could also be a possible hereditary cause. Parents with allergies and food intolerances tend to give birth to children with allergies and intolerances, but whether this is passed on through the genes or the placenta via the blood is not known.

Stress can increase allergies and food intolerances. People who feel stressed often, look for reasons causing the stress and may blame it entirely on their relationships or the work environment. When the diet is altered, frequently stress decreases considerably. Quite often when you feel stressed, you should think about your diet rather than look for the things in your life that cause you stress.

Certain foods can exacerbate stress. Caffeine, for example, can cause anxiety, palpitations, irritability, and insomnia, and food additives have been proved to cause hyperactivity.

In the past, germs have determined the pattern of illness in our society. Today, this is still true, but we have entered an era of human-made illness in which allergies and food intolerances are increasingly prevalent.

The symptoms of a food intolerance

All manner of symptoms may be the result of a food intolerance, ranging from headaches and migraine, chronic fatigue, fluctuating weight, digestive problems, pains in the neck, joints and muscles, arthritis, asthma, eczema, poor concentration and dizziness, to mood swings, emotional outbursts and even violent behavior (also see chart on page 14). In addition, it has been found that food intolerances can be one of the causes of many chronic conditions such as chronic fatigue syndrome, AIDS, and cancer, due to the depletion of the immune system.

The symptoms can also change. An elderly woman suffering from arthritis, for example, may have had constant feeding problems, colicky pains, constipation, and teething troubles in early childhood. She may have suffered from eczema, hay fever, catarrh, repeated coughs, colds and ear infections, and was perhaps hyperactive and had learning and coordination difficulties at school. Later on in her life, she may have suffered from migraines, headaches, asthma, acne, and depression. She may also have been affected by hormonal changes, particularly at puberty, during pregnancy, postnatally, or during menopause. This would have given rise to PMS, heavy or irregular periods, morning sickness during pregnancy, and postnatal and menopausal depression.

Of course, some of the symptoms listed on page 14 may be due to other causes. Insomnia, for example, could be due to a specific incident, which is causing you stress; or a backache may be due to poor seating at work. But if you're experiencing many of these symptoms frequently and severely, and not always for any apparent reason, you'll probably find that allergies and/or intolerances are the cause. So take note if you have inexplicable panic attacks, for example, or if you feel irritable for no reason or have any other persistent problem. For by discovering your allergies and/or intolerances, you may discover the reason for such symptoms.

Symptoms that indicate a food intolerance

- Overweight, underweight, fluctuating weight.
- Itching or burning skin, eczema, urticaria, dandruff, acne, varicose veins.
- Cramps, nausea, vomiting, diarrhea, constipation, bloating, flatulence, colitis, ulcerative colitis, irritable bowel, colic, indigestion, anemia.
- Discomfort in the muscles of the neck.
- Backache, aching muscles or joints, fibrositis, arthritis, tingling in the muscles.
- Insomnia, waking in the night, poor sleep patterns.
- Impaired energy, chronic fatigue.
- Weeping/itching eyes, visual problems, sensitivity to bright lights.
- Sneezing, sinusitis, runny nose, polyps, post-nasal drip, hay fever, nosebleeds.
- Ringing in the ears, earache.
- Sore throat, hoarseness, cough, catarrh, asthma, wheezing, bronchitis, breathlessness.
- Cold/hot sweating extremities, chilblains, hot flushes.
- Fast/slow pulse, high/low blood pressure, palpitations, unexplained anginal pain.
- Dark puffy circles under eyes, constant bruising.
- Painful irregular periods, PMS, thrush.
- Frequent urination, bed-wetting, water retention, cystitis, frequent colds or infections, excessive sweating, low blood sugar.
- Inexplicable fatigue, sleepiness, drowsiness after meals, waking up tired, sleepwalking, nightmares, hallucinations.
- Persistent tension/anxiety/nervousness, panic attacks, poor tolerance to pain.
- Headaches, migraine, convulsions, blackouts, vertigo, dizzy spells, poor coordination.
- Mental confusion, poor concentration, forgetfulness, depression, blank mind, difficulty making decisions.

- Hyperactivity, irritability, aggressiveness, violence.
- Delayed crawling/walking/talking, learning disabilities.
- Colic, fretfulness, earaches, croup.
- Inability to delay or miss a meal, obsessional eating, craving a special food, constant snacking, poor appetite.
- Feeling unwell when food or drink are missed.
- Feeling immediately better after obtaining the food to which one is sensitive.
- Tender or bleeding gums, mouth ulcers, cracks in lips, sore tongue.
- White marks on the nails; splitting nails; discoloration on the skin; dry, flaky skin that's pale in color.
- Excessive hair loss, prematurely gray hair.
- Little desire for sex.
- Infertility.

Detecting allergies and food intolerances

Detecting allergies and food intolerances can be complicated, but if you follow the Elimination Diet in this book, you should find most, if not all, of the answers. Or, you could have your allergies or food intolerances tested at a natural health clinic. In this case, it is worth bearing in mind, that "allergy tests" are not always accurate and that allergies and intolerances can change or increase. A period of general ill health, a viral infection, or any increased stress in your life can lead to an increase in allergic responses. Furthermore, assessing your own problems will give you more control over your body. So you may decide that you want to follow the Elimination Diet before embarking on the Rotation Diet.

chapter 2
preparing
for your diet

The diets in this book cannot be followed halfheartedly. If they are to be successful, it is important to take time to plan and prepare. You need time to collect the new foods you are going to use and to find shops to supply you.

Choose a quiet time of the year to embark on your diet, away from Christmas, festive occasions, or anniversaries when it could be difficult to stick to your regime. For the week prior to starting and during the time you are on either of the diets, you will need to keep a food diary. Make a list on the left side of the page of everything that passes your lips, including drinks and snacks. On the right-hand side, write down any reactions or feelings you experience, and record on a scale of 1 to 10 the severity of these reactions.

Upon starting, it is very important not to include anything else in your diet. Alcohol, coffee, strong tea, cocoa, cola, chocolate, spices or other stimulants, including tobacco, increase any adverse response that may be occurring. This is particularly important when following the Elimination Diet.

This may seem difficult and time-consuming. However, the benefits to your health and to your life will far exceed any minor difficulties you may encounter. As long as you take the time to buy

avoid all unnecessary tablets. Also avoid all vitamins and minerals, as they contain fillers and other hidden substances that could interfere with the diet. If any of your prescription tablets are sugar coated, you can wash the sugar off.

■ Choose long or short grain, organically grown wholemeal rice, obtainable from health-food stores or some supermarkets. The rice should be rinsed thoroughly before using, and you may want to soak the rice in mineral water for 6 to 8 hours prior to cooking. This brings it "alive" and makes it more nutritious.

■ Use green, brown, or puy lentils, but as red lentils have been processed these will not sprout. They are only good for very

The soaking and sprouting of beans, grains, and seeds

Alfalfa, linseeds, fenugreek, sesame, pumpkin, sunflower, and oats will need at least 6 hours' soaking time. Beans, almonds, and other nuts; wheat, rice, millet, and rye will need at least 12 hours.

Special bean sprouters may be purchased for this purpose, but using a jam jar can be just as simple and effective.

1   Take a handful of beans, wash thoroughly, and place in a jam jar. Cover with about three times as much water. Place a piece of muslin or screen over the top for draining, and leave to soak overnight.

2   Rinse and drain through the muslin top, and place the jar, on its side, in a dark, airy cupboard. Repeat this twice a day for 3 to 5 days.

3   On the last 2 days, place the jar in the sunlight, keeping the beans moist while they grow green with chlorophyll.

Refrigerate in a covered container, and use raw in salads, soups, etc. It is advantageous to sprout all beans for 2 to 3 days prior to cooking. Many people who may have difficulty digesting beans will find them acceptable when prepared in this way.

young children or anyone who is unable to cope with the high fiber content in sprouted lentils. Sprouting greatly enhances the nutrient value and digestibility of these foods. Many beans, grains, seeds, and even some nuts will sprout. When water is added, many of the enzyme and metabolic inhibitors that are designed to keep the seed from germinating until the allotted time are washed out. If ingested, these can block our absorption of calcium, zinc and other minerals. The water also activates the germination process and starts the pre-digestion of the proteins, fats, and carbohydrates into amino acids, fatty acids, and simple carbohydrates, respectively. The synthesis of many vitamins also takes place, including vitamin B-complex, C, and E, and these, together with the mineral content, increase immensely.

- The best way to cook vegetables is to steam or boil them in a little water. Any leftover water can be used as stock or simply drunk, as it will contain many of the nutrients.
- Avoid all foods containing additives, preservatives, and colorings, including margarine. Although we need to have plenty of polyunsaturated oil in our diet, margarine is not a good source.
- Polyunsaturated oils contain fatty acids that are essential for health, but these can only be found in certain unrefined and cold pressed oils, as the refining process can turn the fatty acids into harmful trans-fatty acids. Oils should be purchased in glass bottles and refrigerated once opened, as any oil or fat can become rancid when exposed to light or air for any length of time.
- Take great care when cooking with oil. Both fats and oils can produce very toxic substances if overheated or if exposed to light or air for any length of time. This is why lower temperatures have been used in the recipes. Butter or ghee, pure lard (organic), tropical fats (coconut, palm kernel), sesame, and olive oil in this order, produce the least amount

of toxic substances when heated. If you do need to fry, you can cool-fry by putting a little water into the pan with the fat or oil. When using a wok, use a little water rather than oil.

- Check expiration dates, and avoid all sauces and composite foods, e.g., sausages, burgers, etc.

- Do also allow your diet to be as varied as possible. The wealth of whole foods available means that you can eat delicious, exciting meals without having to smother the food in additive-filled sauces. Instead, you will find that you soon begin to appreciate the more subtle and natural flavors of the foods.

- Whenever possible, sit down and eat in a peaceful and settled atmosphere, and give mindful attention to the food you are eating. "Energy flows where attention goes," so your digestion and appreciation of the food will be greatly enhanced if you do this. Try to chew well and avoid reading newspapers over a meal, watching television, eating on the run, or anything else that causes stress on the body.

- Most of the recipes in this book are designed for four people, as this is the average family size. Even though only one member of the family may be following the diet, it will be of great help to that person if the rest of the family eats the same meal, all of whom will benefit.

- Most important, use love, care, and goodwill when preparing and cooking food. The best food can be marred and ruined for everyone if prepared in a hectic or negative frame of mind.

Some of the foods you may want to buy for your kitchen

Agar This is a seaweed-based setting agent similar to gelatine. It is rich in protein and calcium and is easy to digest. It may be bought as granules or flakes. The granules are more processed but stronger. To make, use 1 tsp granules to 1 cup of liquid. With the flakes, use 1 tbsp to 1 cup of liquid. For both types, mix the agar with some or all of the liquid, bring to the boil and simmer for one minute. It sets quickly but may be reheated to liquefy without spoiling.

Amaranth

A relatively new cereal in our stores and useful for highly sensitive people who are unlikely to have built up an intolerance to it. It is gluten free, contains all of the eight amino acids, and is also rich in iron. It is similar to millet in appearance and can be cooked in the same way. Due to its comparatively high protein content, it is also a useful food for vegans who are intolerant to nuts.

Barley

The major grain used in the manufacture of alcohol. It is a glutinous cereal and can be bought as a flour, flakes, as pearl barley, or pot barley. As pearl barley has been processed, it will not sprout, so it is better to buy pot barley.

Buckwheat

A gluten- and wheat-free seed that can be cooked and treated like rice. It is rich in potassium and lysine, an amino acid that most grains lack. It also contains rutin, which is good for strengthening the blood capillaries, helps improve circulation, and stabilizes blood pressure.

Dairy foods

Allergies and intolerances to cow's milk products are extremely common, but the protein in goat's and sheep's milk is more easily digested. Live yogurt, preferably sheep's or goat's, and some cheeses in which the milk has been partially broken down by enzyme action are often tolerated more easily by many. Both goat's and sheep's milk will freeze, although goat's milk can have a somewhat "goaty" flavor unless it is very fresh. Clarified butter can often be tolerated by milk-sensitive people. This is because the milk protein has been separated. It can be bought as "ghee" at Indian food shops and at most supermarkets or can be made at home. To make, melt a pack of butter over gentle heat, allow to cook slightly, and then pour off carefully into a glass jar. The proteins in the butter will have settled on the bottom of the pan. Ghee and butter are the most stable fats for use in cooking.

Flax seed oil (linseed oil)

One of the richest and most stable sources of omega-3 fatty acids. It can be used on salads or taken by the spoonful, 1–2 tbsp a day, but it is not suitable for cooking.

Hemp seed/oil

Hemp is one of the sturdiest and fastest growing plants on the planet, and a plant favored by environmentalists. Its long-penetrating roots draw minerals buried deep in the soil up to the surface, enriching the soil on which it grows and requiring no pesticides, herbicides, and little fertilizer. Hemp seeds are rich in magnesium, potassium, sulphur, and other key elements and contain all the essential amino acids in an easily digestible form. They contain the richest known source of essential fatty acids in their oil and in the perfect ratio for human nutritional needs. The drug tetrahydracannabinol is contained in the leaves and the flowers of certain strains of the hemp plant, and it is for this reason that growing hemp is illegal. However, the drug is not present in the seeds, which are legal and obtainable. They are best eaten raw or ground and made into butters. They can be also added to flours to make hemp breads, etc.

Kamut

An ancient, nonhybridized grain now being produced in the United States and slowly coming to the market in Great Britain that many "wheat-allergic" people can tolerate. It is a variety of high-protein, low-gluten wheat with kernels two to three times the size of wheat grains. Because of its low gluten content, though, it is not so good for making bread.

Kelp

A natural seaweed product that is extremely high in minerals and trace elements, particularly iodine. It may be used as a substitute for salt.

Millet Gluten-free but cheaper to buy than the other grains mentioned and obtainable at most stores. It is the most alkaline of the grains and contains all but one of the essential amino acids. It also contains potassium, iron, and magnesium and is an excellent source of silicon, which is a mineral essential for healthy bones, teeth, nails, and hair. Millet is particularly good for the health and function of the stomach, spleen, and pancreas. Cook like rice, using 1 cup of millet to 2 cups of water, and cook for 25 minutes.

Miso A Japanese seasoning paste similar to yeast extracts in taste and color. It is made from fermented rice, barley, or soy beans, so check the labeling carefully when buying. It is an excellent source of nutrients and is useful as a flavoring for soups and stews.

Olive oil Rich in monounsaturates, though low in essential fatty acids, the cold-pressed, virgin olive oil is the only unrefined oil sold on the mass market. Due to its relative stability and to the ease with which it can be extracted, i.e., it does not require high-pressure pressing equipment, many of its health-giving properties remain intact. It contains vitamin E, phytosterols, chlorophyll, magnesium, carotene, and other beneficial minor ingredients unique to olives. Use virgin olive oil on salads, stirring into vegetables and soups, and for low-temperature cooking as well.

Pepper Black and white pepper can be used on cold or warm food. However, it is important not to heat it or add it to very hot food as it then becomes an irritant to the intestinal mucosa.

Legumes (dried peas, beans, and lentils) These are a good source of protein and fiber. When mixed with a grain such as rice, they provide a complete protein meal, i.e., one that contains all the essential amino acids. It is recommended that these are sprouted for 2 to 3 days prior to cooking, or for 3 to 5 days for eating raw, as this will increase their nutrient value greatly, enhance their digestibility, and reduce cooking time.

Quinoa

Can be used in the same way as millet. It contains all eight essential amino acids and is extremely rich in calcium and iron. It can be cooked in the granule form, or the seeds can be ground to a flour in a blender or coffee grinder.

Rice

One of the oldest cultivated grains. Generally speaking, it is a safe food for most people, but those who have used it as a staple food for many years may need to check carefully for any intolerance. Choose organically grown, short- or long-grain varieties. Whole-grain, basmati, wild, and whole-grain noodles are also available in health food stores. Vermicelli (white Chinese noodles) may be useful in some recipes. Always wash rice grains before cooking. Soaking for 6 to 8 hours prior to cooking will "bring the rice alive" and reduce cooking time.

Safflower, soy bean, and sunflower seed oil

These oils are highly nutritious and rich in polyunsaturates and essential fatty acids but only when unrefined and cold pressed. Use in salads and add to soups and vegetables when raw. If you do need to use these oils in baking, keep the temperature of the oven to below 325°F.

Sesame seed oil

Should be unrefined, untoasted, and cold pressed. In this state, it is a rich source of omega-6 essential fatty acids. Use cold, sprinkled on salads. It remains reasonably stable when heated, so it can be used for low-temperature cooking.

Sorghum

An African grain now grown in many other parts of the world. It is similar in composition to corn, but higher in protein and is available at some health-food stores or by mail order.

Spelt flour

An ancient precursor of modern-day wheat, usually grown organically and often more easily tolerated.

Sweet potatoes, yams, eddoes, and dasheen

Available in most large supermarkets and are sold at many West

Indian food stores. They are all high in carbohydrates and may be used like potatoes. It is also possible to buy sweet potato and yam flours. The flesh of the sweet potato is either whitish or orange, and due to its sweet flavor, can be used in sweet or savory cooking.

Tahini A nut butter made from roasted ground sesame seeds and oil and used as a spread, topping, in dips and dressings, sauces, and soups.

Tamari A naturally produced, wheat-free soy sauce.

Tempeh Cultured from cooked, split soy beans in a similar way to cheese.

Tofu A high-protein, low-fat curd made from soy milk. Both tofu and tempeh are very digestible.

Tropical oils Unrefined and cold pressed palm oil or coconut oil is much more stable when heated than any of the polyunsaturated oils and therefore more suitable for cooking purposes. If you are able to obtain them, you can use them instead of sunflower and safflower oils in recipes.

Umeboshi plums Japanese plums that have been picked green and pickled in brine with shiso (perilla) leaves, which give them the pink color. They are rich in enzymes and are a good digestive aid. They may be bought at health-food stores, whole, and also as a purée.

Walnut oil An excellent source of omega-6 and a smaller amount of omega-3 essential fatty acids as long as it is unrefined and cold pressed.

Wheat Contains gluten, but when the grains are sprouted, the gluten and glutenlike substances found in rye, barley, and oats are broken down by the enzyme action. You may, therefore, find that you can tolerate wheat and similarly, rye, barley, and oats when they are sprouted. In addition, some people find that they can tolerate durum wheat found in wheat pasta, couscous, bulgur wheat, and semolina more easily than the strong wheat flour used in baking. Bread made with French flour may also be an alternative. Wheat seems to absorb more of the pesticides and artificial fertilizers used in farming than other grains, so it is important to buy organically grown wheat.

Wheat germ oil One of the richest sources of vitamin E, and may also protect the heart and help nerve regeneration. Many people, intolerant to the wheat grain, find that they can tolerate wheat germ oil. Take by the spoonful, or cold, on salads.

Choose foods that are natural, whole, pure, and unprocessed; buy organic produce and meat from animals that have been reared in humane conditions, wherever possible. This will reduce the amount of drugs and chemicals you are ingesting.

Adapting the diets to your needs
By following the diets in this book, you will be restricting what you eat for several months. During this time, you may want to alter the diets, and you will also need to consider what to do when away from home, eating out in restaurants, or when traveling.

Case study
Patricia, age 35, heard she could lose weight by avoiding certain foods. Following a test for food intolerances, she was advised to avoid wheat and sugar. After a period of withdrawal symptoms, she began to lose weight slowly. She was then advised to avoid dairy products, soy, peanuts, hazelnuts, and chemical sweeteners. This produced the desired result. She lost 25 pounds. Her friends and family were amazed at the change in her weight and health.

If you work full-time or travel around a lot, these diets should prove to be easy to follow as long as you are prepared. If you make your meals the night before or in the morning, you can pack them into a container and take them with you. There is a tendency to think of sandwiches when it comes to packed lunches. However, that means missing out on all the other things that could go into a lunchbox. Many of the meat dishes and nut roasts are delicious cold, and you can make up rice or millet salads with plenty of raw vegetables, nuts, and seeds. A Thermos of soup is also a good idea.

We are all social beings, and it is important that you do not curtail social engagements because of your new diet. Likewise, it may be tempting to abandon your regime to conform with everyone else. It is simply not worth it. As your health improves, you will notice that your confidence increases, and you will cease to waste time and energy worrying about what others may think.

Eating in restaurants is not usually too much trouble either. If you know what you are looking for, you can usually find food sufficient for your needs. You can ask for the meat or fish without the sauce, for example, and fresh fruit for dessert. Try to resist fried food, as the oil will have been overheated and usually reused. As for a drink, there is always mineral water. Do not be afraid to ask for something different; chefs are often only too willing to oblige.

If you are traveling by plane, airlines will provide special diets without any problem if you remember to state what you want (within reason) at the time you book your ticket.

Dinner parties could prove a little more awkward, but only if you let them. You can tell your host at the time of the invitation that you are following a new diet and you are avoiding certain foods. If this is a problem, you can simply offer to take your own food.

If you have the occasional lapse with the rotation of foods, you can always make adjustments and get back to your routine. It is important to go about the diet as naturally and as calmly as you can. Try not to become overobsessed or too fanatical, as this will lead to a situation where the diet is controlling you rather than your being in charge of it.

The food families

For the diets in this book, you need to be aware of the different food families. This is important because people often react to the "relatives" of the food to which they are intolerant. For instance, if you are reacting to tomato, you may also react to potato, green pepper, chilies and aubergine. In the case of the grass family, to which most cereals belong, we look more to the subdivisions. Many people only react to wheat or corn, the most commonly eaten cereals, for example, or to the cereals that contain gluten or gluten-related substances, namely wheat, rye, barley, and possibly oats.

The food family chart

Apple apples, pears, quince, loquat, pectin, cider.

Arum dasheen, eddoes.

Aster lettuce, endive, globe and Jerusalem artichokes, dandelion, sunflower, salsify, tarragon, chamomile, yarrow, safflower oil.

Banana bananas, plantains, arrowroot.

Beech chestnuts.

Beef beef, veal, all cow's milk products.

Beet sugar beet, spinach, Swiss chard, beets, quinoa.

Birch filberts, hazelnuts, birch oil (wintergreen).

Bird all fowl and game birds, including chicken, turkey, duck, goose, pigeon, quail, pheasant, partridge, grouse, eggs.

Blueberry blueberry, bilberry, cranberry.

Buckwheat buckwheat, rhubarb, sorrel, amaranth (nearest family).

Cashew cashews, pistachios, mangoes.

Citrus lemons, oranges, grapefruits, limes, tangerines, citron.

Conifer juniper, pine nuts.

Crustacean crab, crayfish, lobster, prawn, shrimp.

Freshwater fish salmon, trout, pike, perch, bass.

Fungus mushrooms, yeast.

Ginger East Indian arrowroot, ginger, cardamom, turmeric.

Gooseberry currants, gooseberries.

Grape grapes, raisins, wine, cream of tartar.

Grass wheat, spelt wheat, corn, oats, barley, rye, rice, malt, millet, bamboo shoots, sugar cane, sorghum, kamut.

Honeysuckle elderberry.

Laurel avocadoes, cinnamon, bay leaves.

Lily onions, garlic, asparagus, chives, leeks.

Mallow okra, hibiscus.

Melon watermelon, cantaloupe and other melons, cucumbers, zucchini, marrow, pumpkin, acorn squash and other squashes.

Mint apple mint, basil, bergamot, hyssop, lavender, lemon balm, marjoram, oregano, peppermint, rosemary, sage, spearmint, savory, thyme.

Mollusc abalone, snail, squid, clam, mussel, oyster, scallop, octopus.

Morning glory sweet potatoes.

Mulberry figs, mulberry, hops, breadfruit.

Amaranth*

Buckwheat*

Kelp*

Millet*

Quinoa*

Sorghum*

Sweet potatoes, yams, cassava, eddoes, and dasheen*

Tahini*

Tapioca comes from the cassava root and is sold as pearls, flakes, or as a flour, and can be bought in most supermarket stores. It consists almost entirely of starch, with traces of calcium and other minerals. It can be used in puddings and as a thickener in soups and sauces.

Tiger nuts tubers rather than nuts and about the size of peanuts. They are cultivated in Spain and are available at some health-food stores. They can be used for making "nut" milks and for eating raw as a snack.

Guidelines to help you through the Preliminary Diet

■ Vegetables can be washed in tap water and then rinsed in mineral water. Remember to clean your teeth with mineral water, and check that your toothpaste does not contain sugar or any other substance you are trying to avoid.

■ It is safer to alternate fruits so that you do not eat the same fruit for more than two days in a row, followed by at least two days without that particular fruit. The same applies to herbs, herb teas, and tea. Use powdered ginger and other spices very sparingly, and only use carob powder in the third week.

■ Also take care with fruit sugar, honey, date syrup, rice syrup and maple syrup. Use very little and alternate them if necessary. Some people who are allergic to pollen may react to honey. Also try to choose honey from bees that are unlikely to have been fed on sugar throughout the winter months, such as honey from Mexico, Argentina and Australia. Cold pressed, organic honey is ideal.

■ If you feel better after three weeks, you can then introduce more foods into your diet following the plan laid out in the Elimination Diet. Start at Day 9 with the introduction of tap water and then continue through until Day 28. You will find that some of the foods in those subsequent days, such as avocado pear for example, will not need to be tested as you will have already included them in the Preliminary Diet. All such foods will be marked with an asterisk so you will be able to recognise them immediately. You can simply introduce these foods into your diet as shown without having to test them.

■ If, however, you do not feel any better and you have checked that you are not reacting to any chemicals or fumes, go to the beginning of the Elimination Diet procedure and start at Day 1.

The following menus are only suggestions. You can use any of the recipes in the following pages as well as those from Days 1 to 8 inclusive in the Elimination Diet.

Suggested menus for the Preliminary Diet

Monday
Breakfast
Rice flake muesli (p.84)

Main meals
Grilled mackerel or flounder with gooseberry sauce served with mashed yam and fresh salad
Quinoa nut roast (p.165) served with fresh salad

Light meals
Lentil soup (p.108) with rice bread (p.209)

Tuesday
Breakfast
Millet and buckwheat muesli (millet and buckwheat flakes, chopped almonds, raisins, dates) with almond milk (p.235)

Main meals
Game bird casserole (p.130) served with green vegetables
Vegetable hash browns (p.90) served with fennel and bean sprout salad (p.199)

Light meals
Cream of cauliflower soup with almonds (p.92)

Wednesday
Breakfast
Millet porridge (see Quinoa porridge, p.81) with fresh banana

Main meals
Lamb burgers (p.136) served with sweet potatoes and green vegetables
Barley, cashew and vegetable loaf (p.162) served with fresh salad

Light meals
Sweet potato and seafood bakes (p.163)
Stuffed mushrooms (p.113)

Thursday
Breakfast
Quinoa porridge (p.81) with Hunza apricots

Main meals
Braised venison with juniper (p.141) served with red-currant sauce (p.196), broccoli, and sweet potatoes
Steamed vegetables (p.190) with millet (p.184)

Light meals
Celery and zucchini soup (p.93)

Friday
Breakfast
Rice porridge (p.83) with fresh pears

Main meals
Red mullet with seasoned rice stuffing (p.153) served with spinach
Millet, lentil, and brazil nut loaf (p.162) served with green vegetables or salad

Light meals
Green split pea soup with broccoli (p.94)

Saturday

Breakfast

Rice porridge (p.83) with fresh raspberries

Main meals

Rabbit hot pot (p.133) served with fresh green vegetables

Parsnip and walnut croquettes (p.186) served with raw salad or steamed vegetables

Light meals

Celery and chestnut soup (p.93)

Sunday

Breakfast

Fresh melon with ginger

Main meals

Wild duck with pineapple (p.128) served with sweet potatoes and cauliflower

Apricot and almond pilaf (p.166) with fresh salad

Light meals

Cream of carrot and celery root soup (p.95)

chapter 4 the elimination diet

This diet consists of a modified fast for four days, followed by a gradual reintroduction of foods. Fasting ensures that the digestive system is rested so the body can begin to extract toxins from the cells and tissues. A pure fast would consist of taking nothing by mouth except spring water. Many people do this regularly because it makes them feel good. However, as the purpose of this diet is simply to clear your body of any possible items that may be causing adverse reactions, you do not need to eliminate all foods. Instead, you can eat foods that are very unlikely to cause any reaction and therefore toxins. Only those people familiar with fasting should attempt a water-only fast, as it can release toxins very quickly, often causing intense reactions.

By giving your body time to rest by fasting and cleansing, any food intolerances will start to become "unmasked." One of the effects of this is that any reaction to a food when reintroduced will be more acute, so foods that had little or no apparent effect on you may suddenly produce noticeable reactions. It will therefore be easy for you to work out whether a food is causing any problems. Whereas before, your body may have reacted only when run-down or under stress, and therefore less able to cope, the clearer your body becomes, the more definite the signs will be. You will also find that you can start to listen to your body and sense what it is telling you. This is an important first step to full health.

Do not be put off by the thought of having to change your daily life. Simply go about the alterations methodically and positively. Once you have bought the necessary items for your kitchen and cupboard (see page 23) and eliminated the things that need to be eliminated, you can then just incorporate the changes into your routine. The difference this can make to your health and to your life can be wonderful.

Withdrawal symptoms

During the first four days of the Elimination Diet, you are likely to feel unwell due to withdrawal symptoms, but by Day 5 you should feel better and will be able to start the reintroduction of foods, as suggested here.

Foods are reintroduced according to their food family. When you test the foods, you will be able to tell whether or not you are allergic or intolerant to them. If you react to any foods, you should then avoid them. The recipes have been designed to make this as easy as possible for you. If you do not react, you can then simply introduce them into your diet as the plan shows you. You may notice that some foods will not be introduced into the diet immediately after testing. This is simply a precaution in case you react more slowly to them as people sometimes do. The majority of foods, though, will produce immediately recognizable symptoms.

Symptoms might vary from food to food. Some foods will produce more severe reactions, and others, more delayed ones. The types of symptoms can also differ enormously. Sometimes, for example, you may experience panic attacks, other times just a faint headache. This is where the pulse test is invaluable (see page 18). Do not forget to use this and then to record all reactions in your food diary (see page 16).

Guidelines to help you through the Elimination Diet

◼ If you can, try to test the foods in as many different ways as possible – raw, lightly cooked, and cooked slowly for a longer time, as this may make a difference as to whether or not you react. The recipes and the menus have been designed to help you to do this. Do not worry, though, if you cannot test all the members of each food family (see page 31). There are, of course, exceptions to the rule, but normally if you react to one member of a family, you will do so to all the others. Those that are the normal exceptions have been introduced separately into the 28-day plan.

◼ For those with multiple food intolerances, it may be that you will need to slow down the diet a little. For some people, just introducing one new food or food family at a time will be sufficient. Remember that this is a diet about getting well, not about racing to the end. If you are unsure about a reaction, you can leave the food family out and test again in four days' time.

◼ You may find that you are trying out new foods that you have not eaten before. This is a good idea, not only because it offers you delicious new foods but it will also mean your diet may not be as limited as it might if you have to start avoiding certain foods. So try the quail eggs, the venison,

---

Case study

Sandra was always in trouble at school. She fell asleep over her desk, never did her homework, and frequently arrived late. Her school demanded that Sandra see a psychologist, who suggested that she was taking "social" drugs. Her parents knew this was wrong, however, and decided to check for allergies instead. Sandra was found to be reacting to milk products, corn, potatoes, tomatoes, tea, and particularly car fumes. Steps were taken to deal with all this, and Sandra never fell asleep at school again.

the allergy exclusion diet

and the tiger nuts, for example. They are delicious, and a way of ensuring you do not feel you are depriving yourself.

■ Once you have completed the Elimination Diet, you will have discovered which foods you are reacting to, and you can avoid these items so your system can have a rest. In this way it will have a chance to recover and rebalance. You may want to make a list of all the foods you have had a reaction to and note the severity of the reaction. If the reaction was only a minor one, you may find that you can eat it on an occasional basis, perhaps once a week, or in the following Rotation Diet. Foods that cause major reactions, though, will need to be avoided for two to three months before being tested again.

The 28-day Elimination Diet plan

DAY 1
Rice
Pears
Lamb or lentils

DAY 2
Rice
Pears
Lamb or lentils

DAY 3
Rice
Pears
Lamb or lentils
Equisetum tea

DAY 4
Rice
Pears
Lamb or lentils
Linden leaf tea

DAY 5
Rice
Lamb
Mustard family
Kiwi fruit
Flaxseed oil
  (linseed)

DAY 6
Quinoa
Fish: Oily saltwater
Sweet potatoes
Arum family
Mallow family
Melon family
Gooseberry family
Olive oil
Mint family tea
Fruit sugar

DAY 7
Buckwheat family
Millet, tapioca
Game bird
Walnut family
Tiger nuts
Parsley family
Banana family
Pineapples, papayas
Walnut oil
Fennel tea
Maple syrup

DAY 8
Sago
Sorghum
Yam
Rabbit, hare
Aster family
Plum family
Sunflower oil
Safflower oil
Almond oil
Honey
Chamomile tea

DAY 9
Rice
Lamb
Tap water
Pea family
  (not soy)
Pears, quince,
  loquat, lychees
Brazil nuts
Macadamia nuts
Lemon verbena tea
Fenugreek tea

DAY 10
Barley
Fish: Saltwater
Venison
Beet family, olives
Rose family
Conifer family
Pumpkin seeds
Mulberry family
Cashew family
Lemongrass tea
Raspberry leave tea

DAY 11
Quail, quail's eggs
Lily family
Laurel family
Citrus family
Blueberry family
Chestnuts
Birch family
Taheebo Tea
  (Pau Darco)
Orange juice
Rice syrup

DAY 12
Beef and veal
Potato family
Grape family
Seaweed
Palm family
Sesame seeds
  and oil
Date syrup

DAY 13
Pork, wild boar
Soy products
Mushrooms
Apples, pectin
Mustard seed

DAY 14
Oats
Fish: freshwater
Ginger family
Nutmeg family

DAY 15
Turkey
Rooibosch tea
Myrtle family
Black and white
   pepper

DAY 16
Corn
Chicory coffee
Dandelion coffee
Barleycup

DAY 17
Yeast
Green leaf tea

DAY 18
Rye
Fish: crustacean
   family

DAY 19
Duck, goose
Duck's eggs,
   goose eggs

DAY 20
Sheep's milk
   products

DAY 21
Cane sugar
Wine vinegar

DAY 22
Wheat, spelt wheat
Kamut
Fish: mollusk
   family

DAY 23
Chicken
Chicken's eggs

DAY 24
Goat's milk
   products

DAY 25
Tea
Peanuts
Cider vinegar

DAY 26
Cocoa

DAY 27
Coffee

DAY 28
Cow's milk
   products

Days 1 to 4

Eat any of the following:

Pears

Rice

Lamb or lentils

Sea salt

Mineral water

Equisetum (horsetail) and **linden leaf tea** on Days 3 and 4.

- If you suffer from arthritis, you may find that red meat is too acidic for you, in which case you may want to avoid lamb altogether and substitute lentils or maybe the mustard family.
- **It is very important to exclude everything else from your diet.** A small drink of tea or coffee could alter the whole experiment and you would need to start again. This also includes smoking. This may seem extreme, but it is worth persevering. The diet is for a relatively short amount of time, and it can bring a lifetime's benefit.

Suggested menu

Upon rising

Drink 2 glasses of hot water

8am   1 to 2 fresh pears

10am   Grilled lamb or a serving of lentils and rice

1pm   Lamb with rice or lentils with rice

4pm   Fresh pear

6pm   Rice porridge with cooked pears

9pm   Fresh pear

Day 5

Introduce and test the following:

The mustard family: turnip, rutabaga, radish, daikon, watercress, mustard and cress, bok choy, cabbage, cauliflower, broccoli, sprouts, kohlrabi, kale.

Kiwi fruit

Flaxseed oil (linseed oil): This may be sprinkled on salads or added to mashed vegetable, but do not use this oil for cooking. Lamb drippings can be saved for this purpose.

Suggested menu

Breakfast

Fresh pears with rice porridge (p.83)

Vegetable hash browns (p.90)

Main meal

Grilled lamb with green vegetables and mashed rutabaga

Rice and lentils with green vegetables and mashed rutabaga

Light meal

Turnip and watercress soup (p.94)

Steamed vegetables with rice

Raw salad

Sliced bok choy, watercress, mustard and cress, radishes or grated daikon dressed with safflower oil

Fruit

Pears

Kiwi fruit

Drinks

Mineral water

Linden leaf tea

Rice milk (p.234)

Day 6

You now need to come off rice, pears, lentils, and lamb in order to test them on Day 9.

Soak tiger nuts overnight for Day 7.

Introduce and test the following:

Quinoa

Sweet potatoes, dasheens, and eddoes

Fruit sugar

Olive oil

Saltwater fish: mackerel, sardines, herring, fresh tuna, anchovies, halibut, flounder, red or gray mullet.

The mallow family: okra, hibiscus.

The melon family: watermelon, cantaloupe and other melons, cucumbers, zucchini, marrow, pumpkins, acorn squash, and other squashes.

The gooseberry family: gooseberry, red-, white- and black currants.

The mint family: fresh peppermint tea, sage, basil, lemon balm, thyme, rosemary, marjoram, oregano.

Suggested menu

Breakfast

Melon

Quinoa porridge (p.81) with stewed gooseberries or kiwi fruit

Main meal

Grilled sardines with baked sweet potato and cucumber salad

Grilled mackerel, with gooseberry sauce and cucumber salad

Light meal

Sweet potato and seafood bakes (p.163)

Raw salad

Cucumbers and suitable vegetables from the mustard family, and okra

Fruit

Melon

Stewed or raw black currants or gooseberries

Drinks

Mineral water

Peppermint, lemon balm, sage, thyme, rosemary and hibiscus tea.

Day 7

Prepare and soak the lentils and beans today that you wish to use on Day 9.

Introduce and test the following:

Millet

Cassava (tapioca)

Maple syrup

The buckwheat family: buckwheat, rhubarb, sorrel, amaranth.

Wild game bird: pigeon, wild duck, partridge, grouse, pheasant.

Walnuts, pecan nuts, hickory nut, butternut, tiger nuts

Walnut oil

The parsley family: carrots, parsnips, celery, fennel, anise, parsley, caraway, dill, cumin, cilantro, lovage.

The banana family: bananas, plantains, arrowroot.

Pineapple

Papaya

NB: Nuts and seeds can be tested on their own before adding to recipes.

Suggested menu

Breakfast

Diced pineapple and banana fruit salad

Millet porridge (p.81) or Buckwheat muesli (p.85) with pecan nuts, banana and tiger nut milk (p.233)

(Millet and millet porridge can be cooked in the same way as quinoa, or you can use millet flakes. Buckwheat and millet flakes may be used to make up the muesli.)

Main meal

Game bird casserole (p.130) with broccoli, sprouts, or other green vegetables

Parsnip and walnut croquettes (p.186) served with carrots and green vegetables

Light meals

Cream of carrot and celery root soup (p.95)

Celery, walnut, and fennel salad with buckwheat pasta

Grated carrot, celery, and nut salad with millet

Puddings

Baked bananas with chopped pecan nuts and maple syrup

Drinks

Mineral water

Fennel tea

Day 8

Test and introduce the following foods into your diet:

Yam, sago, sorghum

Rabbit, hare

The Aster family: lettuce, endive, salsify, globe and Jerusalem artichokes, dandelions, sunflower seeds, tarragon, chamomile, yarrow.

The Plum family: plums, cherries, peaches, apricots, nectarines, prunes, almonds.

Sunflower, safflower oil and almond oil

Chamomile tea

Honey

Light meals
Baked tomato soup (p.98) with barley scone bread (p.208)
Green pepper and pine nut pizza (p.168) with salad

Day 13

Introduce and test the following:

Soy and soybean products: soy flour, soy milk, soy dried milk, soy oil, soy meat substitutes, tofu, tempeh, soy egg replacer, tamari soy sauce.

Wild boar and outdoor reared pork

Apples and pectin: some sugar-free jams are made with apple juice and pectin.

Mushrooms: including wild porcini, oyster, and shiitake.

*Mustard seed

Suggested menu

Breakfast
Fresh apples
Rice porridge (p.83) with stewed apples and raisins and soy milk (p.236)

Main meal
Wild boar cutlets with mushroom sauce (p.151) served with green beans and yam
Pork, apple, and chestnut pie (soy mince may be substituted for pork) (p.146), served with seasonal vegetables or salad

Light meal
Yellow split pea soup (p.99)
Smoked tofu and mushroom kebabs (p.167) with fresh salad

Day 14

Test **oats** and introduce on Day 16.

Introduce the following:
Freshwater fish: salmon, trout, pike, perch, bass.
***Ginger family**: arrowroot, acrimony, cardamom, ginger, turmeric.
***Nutmeg family:** nutmeg, mace.

Suggested menu
Breakfast
Fresh melon with ground ginger and fruit sugar
Pear and ginger fruit slice (p.89)

Main meals
Fresh salmon with raspberry coulis (p.156) served with rice and green beans
Cardamom nut rice (p.185) with fresh green salad

Light meals
Stuffed papayas (p.187)
Breadfruit with ginger and green peppers (p.169)

Day 15

Introduce and test the following:
Turkey
***The myrtle family**: allspice, cloves, guava.
Black and white pepper: this can be used uncooked, on cold food. When it is cooked, however, pepper can become an irritant and is not good for the liver.
***Rooibosch tea:** this is an African tea available at health-food stores and some supermarkets. It is additive and caffeine free and low in tannin and may be made like ordinary tea and served with a slice of lemon.

You can have quail's eggs again today, but do not use them again until you have tested duck's eggs on Day 19. This is to give you a four-day gap.

Suggested menu
Breakfast
Freshly squeezed orange juice
Buckwheat muesli (p.85) with millet
Poached or scrambled quail's eggs

Main meals
Turkey and mushroom fricassée (p.126) with sautéed sweet potato and fresh green salad (p.198)
Cauliflower and chickpea curry (p.175) with whole-meal basmati rice and sliced tomatoes

Light meals
Onion and barley soup (p.96)
Stuffed baked potato (p.180) with coleslaw (p.201)

Day 16

Test **corn** (corn starch, corn meal, corn flour, sweetcorn), and introduce on Day 18.
You can introduce oats, providing you have not had any adverse reactions.
If you wish, you can introduce barleycup, chicory, and dandelion coffee substitutes. Chicory and dandelion belong to the Aster family.

Suggested menu
Breakfast
Fresh fruit
Oat milk (p.233)
Old-fashioned oatmeal porridge (p.82)
Date and coconut muesli bars (p.218)

Main meals

Shoulder of lamb with raisin, apricot, and oat stuffing (p.138) with new potatoes and seasonal green vegetables

Green pepper and eggplant flan (p.171) served with arame seaweed with sesame seeds (p.199) and fresh green salad (p.198)

Light meals

Miso soup (p.98) with cornbread (p.208)

Hummus and cannellini bean dip (p.118) with crudités

Day 17

Test and introduce **yeast** and **green leaf tea,** which is a china tea, low in caffeine and tannin. It is drunk without milk but may be served with lemon.

Suggested menu

Breakfast

Pears and rice porridge (p.83)

Barley muffins (p.218)

Main meal

Venison steak burgers (p.141) with mixed vegetables and salad

Light meals

Mushroom and black bean soup (p.100)

Rice, barley, and bean sprout salad (p.201)

Day 18

Introduce **corn,** providing you have not had any adverse reactions. Test **rye** and introduce on Day 20.

NB: If you buy rye/pumpernickel bread, check that it does not contain any wheat.

Introduce and test the following:

The crustacean family: crab, crayfish, lobster, prawn, shrimp.

Suggested menu

Breakfast

Fresh melon

Quinoa porridge (p.81) with ginger syrup (p.195)

Main meals

Prawn, avocado, and fennel salad with buckwheat pasta (p.202)

Stuffed green peppers (p.191) served with baby corn and sugar peas

Light meals

Sweetcorn and lima bean succotash soup (p.107) with rye crackers

Open sandwiches using pumpernickel rye bread (p.122)

Day 19

Test **duck and goose** and **duck's eggs and goose eggs,** but do
not introduce duck's eggs into your diet until you have tested
chicken's eggs on Day 23. You can continue to have duck after
today, though, provided you have had no adverse reactions.

Suggested menu

Breakfast

Orange and grapefruit salad

Buckwheat muesli (p.85) with millet

Main meals

Roast duck with orange and grapefruit sauce (p.129) with green
beans or seasonal vegetables

Millet, hazelnut and tofu croquettes (p.193) with tomato sauce
(p.196) served with vegetables

Light meals

Celery and chestnut soup (see page 93)

Stuffed tomatoes (see page 114)

Day 20

Test **sheep's milk products,** but do not introduce into your diet until after Day 28 when you will have tested cow's milk yogurt and cheese.

Rye can now be introduced providing you are clear of any adverse reaction.

Suggested menu
Breakfast
Fresh fruit with sheep's milk yogurt
Rye crackers with sheep's cheese and alfalfa sprouts

Main meals
Creamy lamb with rye spaghetti (p.139)
Fresh green salad
Baked beans in tomato sauce (p.179) served with baked potatoes and fresh green salad

Light meals
Leek and potato soup (p.100) with rye bread (p.211)
Greek salad (p.203)

Day 21

Test **cane sugar,** but do not introduce.
Test and introduce **wine vinegar.**

Suggested menu
Breakfast
Fresh fruit
Compote of mixed dried fruit (figs, prunes, pears, apricots) with rolled oats

Main meals

Pork tenderloin with prune, anchovy, and almond stuffing (p.147)
served with rice, carrots, and peas
Sweet and sour vegetables/pork (p.148) served with basmati
wholemeal rice

Light meals

Green split pea soup with broccoli (p.94)
Stuffed mushrooms (p.113)

Day 22

Test **wheat** (spelt wheat and kamut if available), and introduce
in 2 days' time on Day 24 providing you have had no adverse
reactions. **Spelt wheat** is an ancient precursor of modern-day
wheat and is often more easily tolerated. **Kamut** is an ancient,
nonhybridized grain, now being produced in the United States
and slowly coming to the market in Great Britain. It is a variety
of high-protein, low-gluten wheat. It is usually tolerated well by
"wheat-allergic" people.

Introduce and test following:
The mollusk family: abalone, snail, squid, clams, mussels, oysters,
scallops, octopus.

Suggested menu
Breakfast
Fresh fruit
Lamb burgers (p.136)

Main meals
Seafood paella (p.160) with fresh green salad
Vegetable and lentil dal (p.174) with bulgur wheat (p.191)
(for testing) or millet

Light meals
Spiced pumpkin and ginger soup (p.104) with organic whole-meal bread (for testing)
Tortillas with sweetcorn and tomato filling (p.116) served with fresh green salad

Day 23
Introduce and test **chicken** and **chicken's eggs**. Providing you have not experienced any adverse reactions, you can now use all eggs including quail's and duck's in your diet.

Suggested menu
Breakfast
Fresh fruit
Tropical fruit muesli
Boiled egg

Main meal
Curried chicken (p.125) with rice, buckwheat chapatis (p.212) and sliced tomatoes or pineapple chunks
Sweet potato and parsnip bakes (p.176) served with fresh green salad

Light meal
Garden vegetable soup (p.101)
Avocado sweet and sour salad (p.204)

Day 24
Introduce and test **goat's milk products:** goat's milk, cheese and live yogurt.

Suggested menu
Breakfast
Fresh fruit with goat's milk yogurt
Scrambled egg on toast

Main meals

Chili con carne (p.145) served with long-grain rice and fresh green salad (p.198)

Lamb or vegetable moussaka (p.140) with fresh green salad (p.198)

Light meals

Cream of artichoke soup (p.101)

Day 25

Test **tea** and **cider vinegar**. You can also test **peanuts,** but take care not to eat too many because they may contain carcinogenic substances made by a fungus to which they are very susceptible.

Suggested menu

Breakfast

Fresh apple, pear, or lychees

Corn flakes (organic) with soy or nut milk (pages 230–236)

Main meals

Fruit-roasted leg of wild boar (p.152) with mashed potatoes, baked red cabbage (p.190), and garden peas

Root vegetable crumble (p.177) with baked red cabbage (p.177) and green vegetables

Light meals

Celery and zucchini soup (p.93)

Barley, cashew, and vegetable loaf (p.162) with fennel and bean sprout salad (p.199)

Tofu mayonnaise (p.195)

Day 26

Test **cocoa**. Chocolate bars made from organically grown cocoa beans can be bought at most health-food stores.

Suggested menu

Breakfast

Fresh fruit

Chocolate hazelnut biscuits (p.222)

Main meals

Pot roast leg of lamb (p.137) served with mashed potatoes and broccoli

Kedgeree (p.178) served with fresh spinach and carrots

Millet, lentil, and brazil nut loaf (p.162)

Light meals

Salmon and tomato fish cakes (p.156)

Prawn or tofu chow mein (p.157)

Day 27

Test **coffee**. Use filtered organic coffee (instant coffee contains chemicals). Coffee is a stimulant and can increase any adverse response that may be occurring, so only drink in moderation, if at all.

Suggested menu

Breakfast

Avocado fruit cocktail (p.89)

Sprouted grain bread (p.212)

Main meals

Chicken noodle main meal soup (p.102)

Wild duck with pineapple (p.128) served with braised celery (p.192)

Spanish omelette (p.161) served with boiled potatoes and fresh green salad

Light meals

Broccoli with ginger and macadamia nuts (p.188) served with couscous (or quinoa)

Day 28

Test and introduce the following:

Cow's milk and **cow's milk products**: yogurt, cheese, cream, butter, and ghee (clarified butter). Clarified butter can often be tolerated by milk-sensitive people. This is because the milk protein, traces of which are found in butter, have been separated. It can be bought as ghee at Indian food shops and at most supermarkets. It can also be made at home by melting a pack of butter over gentle heat, allowing it to cook slightly and then pouring off the liquid into a glass jar. The proteins in the butter will then have settled on the bottom of the pan.

Suggested menu

Breakfast

Fresh fruit with organic cow's milk yogurt

Celebration carrot cake (p.214)

Main meals

Lamb noisettes (p.135) with a cheesy rice topping, garnished with mushrooms and served with seasonal green vegetables

Vegetarian/lamb shepherd's pie (p.136) served with green vegetables

Light meals

Minestrone soup (p.103)

Stuffed baked potatoes (p.180) with choice of fillings and fresh green salad (p.198)

chapter 5
the rotation diet

Having established which foods you are reacting to, it is now helpful to follow a Rotation Diet. The purpose of a Rotation Diet is to prevent the development of new allergies and intolerances to foods. Often people find that if they avoid the foods to which they are allergic or intolerant, they experience a great improvement in their health initially but can then start to feel unwell again. This is because they have become allergic or intolerant to something else in the meantime—often a substitute food, which they have eaten too frequently. For example, it is common for someone to replace cow's milk with soy milk, only to find they then develop an intolerance to soy. In addition, a Rotation Diet can also reduce existing food allergies and intolerances, as it allows the body to process each food properly. Hence, it is a way for many people to overcome their intolerances and, for those with multiple food allergies and intolerances, it can often mean they can include more items in their diet than they may otherwise be able to do.

On average, it takes three days for a meal to pass through the human digestive system and to be processed by the body, so to be safe, the diet is based on a four-day plan. For example, if you were to eat wheat on Monday, you would then not have it again until Thursday.

With the exception of the grass family, when foods are rotated, it is the whole food family to which the particular food belongs that is rotated (see page 31). This is important because people can cross-react to the "relatives" of a food to which they are intolerant. For instance, if you are intolerant to onions, you may suspect leeks, garlic, chives, and possibly asparagus. For more information, see pages 31–33.

You will need to avoid foods that you know cause reactions. The recipes have been designed to make it easy for you to leave out any of the foods you cannot tolerate and perhaps substitute other foods that you can. You may also find that as your body clears, small sensitivities that had previously been masked may appear. In this case, you will need to avoid these as well.

However, if you have multiple allergies or intolerances and therefore have a very limited diet, you may have to eat some of the foods that cause the least reactions. If so, it is best to limit these to just once in the particular day. Or, you may find you can tolerate some foods if eaten less frequently—once in eight days, for example.

As the weeks go by and you feel your health improving, you could try to introduce a suspect food into your diet plan. It may very well be that as your body clears, so do your allergies and food intolerances. It is likely then that foods to which you previously reacted may no longer cause you any problems. If this is so, you can simply incorporate the food into your Rotation Diet. As long as you continue to rotate those foods, you should find that they remain safe foods for you.

This diet, therefore, may seem slightly tricky at first, but the benefits are numerous and long-lasting. It is possible to recover your health from an allergy or food-intolerance problem, and a Rotation Diet should prove to be an important part of such a recovery.

Making changes in your diet

Once you have mastered the principles, you may want to rearrange some of the food families. If, for example, you wanted to make a chicken and mushroom pie, you could move the mushrooms from Day 1 to Day 3. You would do this simply by avoiding mushrooms on Day 1 and then having them on Day 3. You then need to wait at least three more days before you could eat them again. If you wanted to move them back to Day 1, you would need to avoid them on the following Day 1 and then reintroduce them on the subsequent Day 1. If you then wanted to switch avocadoes from Day 2 to Day 4, you would need to remember that cinnamon and bay leaves belong to the same family as avocadoes. So you would have to wait until Day 4 before you could eat any of them.

Case study

Jim had suffered from fatigue since the age of nine, which at times turned into complete exhaustion. He had been an athlete in school, but when he became unable to walk very far, he had to stop playing. He then found he could not concentrate and was unable to do his schoolwork. He felt continually ill, as if he had a viral illness. The doctor thought he was depressed and at one point recommended he should leave home and attend a psychiatric center. His parents did not agree with this diagnosis and kept Jim at home. His parents then heard about the work of clinical ecologists in the U.S. and visited a clinic in New York. The advice given was to follow an elimination diet. A lot of vitamin and mineral supplements were also recommended, as well as amino acids, enzymes, and glandular substances. The family started on the diet, and on Day 5, Jim felt much better. He gradually became stronger and began to be able to concentrate. Over the next few months there were several relapses. The family discovered a clinic using clinical ecological methods in England. Each time he relapsed, more foods were found to be causing symptoms. The family was then taught how to plan a rotation diet so that no food was eaten too frequently. This solved a lot of the problems, and Jim was able to study again. In 1989, Jim finished a university degree. During his four years of study, he cooked his own food and kept to a rotation diet. He attended social functions taking his food with him, and then went on to full-time work. Jim realizes that without a knowledge of rotation diets he might still be getting the wrong diagnoses and treatment, and he doubts that he would ever have completed his education.

The 4-day Rotation Diet plan

Day	1	2	3	4
Cereals and grains	Millet Wheat, spelt wheat Barley Rye Kamut	Corn (maize) Oats Sorghum Arrowroot	Rice Wild rice Quinoa Sago flour Any pulse flour	Amaranth Buckwheat Tapioca Chestnut flour
Meat	Rabbit/hare Crustacean family Mollusk family Freshwater fish Yeast	Pork, wild boar Venison	Bird family Eggs	Beef, veal Lamb Saltwater fish Dairy products
Nuts and seeds	Cashew family Sesame	Brazil nuts Pine nuts Macadamia nuts Tiger nuts Pumpkin seeds Hemp seeds	Almonds Coconuts Sunflowers	Hazelnut Chestnut Walnut family Poppyseeds
Sugars	Malt barley Cane sugar	Fruit sugar Corn syrup Oat syrup	Honey Date syrup Beet sugar Rice syrup	Maple syrup Apple/pear concentrate
Drinks	Tea Green leaf tea	Oat milk Hibiscus tea Mint teas Lemon verbena	Soy milk Rice milk Rooibosch tea Cocoa	Sheep's milk Goat's milk Coffee Equisetum tea
Vegetables	Parsley family Seaweed, kelp Mushrooms	Mallow family Melon family Potato family Lily family Laurel family Olives	Aster family Beet family Pea family	Arum family Mustard family Sweet potato Yam Sorrel
Herbs and spices	Parsley family Pepper family	Mint family Ginger family Juniper berries	Tarragon Fenugreek Nutmeg family	Lemongrass Myrtle family Capers
Fruit	Citrus family Blueberry family Mulberry family Elderberry Pomegranate Passion fruit Papaya Mango	Gooseberry family Banana family Pineapple	Kiwi fruit Plum family Dates Cape gooseberries Grape family	Apple family Rose family Guava Lychees Rhubarb
Oils, etc. (should be cold pressed and glass bottled)	Sesame oil Wheat germ oil	Olive oil Hemp seed oil Flaxseed (linseed) oil	Sunflower oil Safflower oil Soy oil Almond oil Tropical oils Wine vinegar Balsamic	Vinegar Walnut oil Hazelnut oil Cider vinegar Raspberry vinegar

Day 1

The following foods can be eaten:

Cereals: wheat, semolina and couscous (wheat), bulgur wheat, spelt wheat flour, kamut, barley, rye, ryevita, pumpernickel bread, millet; wheat, rye, barley, millet and kamut pasta.

Meat, fish etc.: rabbit and hare; the crustacean family (crab, crayfish, lobster, prawn, shrimp); the mollusk family (abalone, snail, squid, clam, mussel, oyster, octopus, scallop); freshwater fish (salmon, trout, pike, perch, bass); barley miso; yeast.

Nuts & seeds: cashew nuts, pistachio nuts; sesame seeds and spread (tahini).

Sugars: barley malt, cane sugar.

Drinks: barley cup, tea, green leaf tea, Maté tea, fennel tea, lime tea, orange juice.

Vegetables: the parsley family (carrots, parsnips, celery, fennel); seaweed, kelp; mushrooms.

Herbs and spices: aniseed, caraway, dill, cumin, cilantro, chervil, fennel leaf or seed.

Fruit: the citrus family (lemons, oranges, grapefruit, limes, tangerines, citron); mangoes, papayas, star fruit, passion fruit, pomegranate; figs, breadfruit, mulberries; cranberries, blueberries; elderberries.

Oils: sesame seed oil, wheat germ oil.

Suggested menus

Breakfasts

Grapefruit and orange fruit salad

Frumenty (p.86)

Millet and kamut porridge (p.82)

Barley flake muesli (p.84)

Grilled trout fillets with tropical fruit (p.90)

Soups and starters

Mushroom and barley broth (p.105)

Parsnip and cilantro soup (p.105)

Clear vegetable and nori broth (p.106)

Fish and fennel soup (p.106)
Pistachio and rabbit/liver pâté (p.111)
Stuffed mushrooms (p.113)

Main meal dishes
Pot roast rabbit with mushroom and fennel stuffing (p.134)
Rabbit/hare hot pot (p.133)
Grilled trout fillets with tropical fruit (p.158)
Stuffed squid (p.159)

Vegetarian main meals
Millet croquettes (p.179)
Barley, cashew, and vegetable loaf (p.162)
Cashew nut and celery flan (p.170)
Mixed vegetable terrine (p.181)

Vegetables and salads
Salad dressing (p.198)
Orange and fennel salad (p.203)
Braised celery (p.192)
Mixed grain salad (p.205)
Seafood salad (p.206)

Puddings and desserts
Fig and lime sorbet (p.224)
Blood oranges with cranberries (p.224)
Pistachio nut semolina with lime (p.225)

Breads, cakes, and biscuits
Soda bread (p.210), Pita bread (p.213)
Sprouted grain bread (p.212)
Barley and cashew nut scones (p.219)
Rye bread (p.211)
Carrot and fig slice (p.221)
Orange and cashew nut crunchies (p.222)

Drinks and miscellaneous
Cashew nut milk (p.234)

Carrot and cashew nut spread (p.237)

Mushroom and tahini spread (p.237)

Lemon and orange barley water (p.230)

Lemon and elderflower cordial (p.2321)

Elderberry punch (p.231)

Day 2
The following foods can be eaten:

Cereals: corn meal, corn flour, corn starch, corn pasta, sorghum, arrowroot, oats, oatmeal, oat cakes, green banana flour.

Meats etc.: pork, wild boar, venison.

Nuts & seeds: Brazil nuts and spread, tiger nuts, macadamia nuts, pine nuts, pumpkin seeds, hemp seeds.

Sugars: fruit sugar, corn syrup, oat syrup.

Drinks: peppermint tea, mint tea, thyme tea, sage tea, lemon verbena and lemon balm tea, black currant leaf tea, hibiscus tea.

Vegetables: avocados, cucumbers, marrow, pumpkins, zucchini, okra, plantain potatoes, tomatoes, eggplant, peppers, onions, leeks, garlic, sweetcorn.

Herbs and spices: cayenne pepper, paprika pepper, ginger, turmeric, cardamom, cinnamon, bay, mint, basil, sage, oregano, thyme, rosemary, lemon balm, chives.

Fruit: bananas, melons, kiwis, currants, gooseberries, pineapples.

Oils: virgin olive oil, flaxseed oil, hemp seed oil.

Suggested menus
Breakfast
Melon salad

Rolled-oat muesli (p.85)

Old fashioned oatmeal porridge (p.82)

Speedy oat porridge (p.81)

Sorghum porridge (p.82)

Polenta (p.86)

Soups and starters

Baked tomato soup (p.98)

Avocado and green pepper soup (p.104)

Spiced pumpkin and ginger soup (p.104)

Gazpacho (p.109)

Tortillas with sweetcorn and tomato filling (p.116)

Avocado and zucchini dip (p.117)

Main meals

Pork and pineapple kebabs (p.149)

Roast pork/wild boar with juniper (p.151)

Pig's liver and onions (p.149)

Venison and cucumber stir-fry (p.142)

Meatballs in tomato sauce (p.150)

Vegetarian main meals

Polenta with tomato and pepper sauce (p.182)

Green pepper and zucchini flan (p.171)

Brazil nut roast (p.164)

Vegetables and salads

Cucumber, avocado, and asparagus salad (p.204)

Greek-style onions (p.189)

Baked plantains (p.193)

Baked vegetables (p.189)

Puddings and desserts

Pineapple upside-down cake (p.214)

Grilled pineapple with macadamia nuts (p.226)

Fruit crêpes (p.226)

Cakes and biscuits

Green banana and oatmeal scones (p.220)

Brazil nut cookies (p.223)

Drinks and miscellaneous

Tiger nut milk (p.233)

Oat milk (p.233)

Hemp seed milk (p.233)

Banana milk shake (p.232)

Brazil nut butter (p.237)

Hemp seed butter (p.238)

Day 3

The following foods can be eaten:

Cereals: brown rice, brown rice flakes, flour and bran, rice pasta, rice cakes, rice biscuits, wild rice, quinoa, quinoa flakes and flour, sago, sago flour, soy flour, lentil flour, gram flour (chickpea), any other legume flour.

Meat, etc.: chicken and eggs, duck and eggs, quail and eggs, turkey, pigeon, and any other game bird, tofu, tempeh, rice or soy miso, Umeboshi plum dressing, Tamari soy sauce.

Nuts & seeds: coconut, almonds, sunflower seeds (not peanuts).

Sugars: honey, rice syrup, date syrup, beet sugar.

Drinks: chicory coffee, dandelion root chip coffee, Rooibosch African tea, soy milk, cocoa, carob, chamomile tea, grape juice.

Vegetables: the aster family (lettuce, endive, globe and Jerusalem artichoke; sunflower seed sprouts); the beet family (beets, spinach, Swiss chard); the pea family (peas, snow peas, sugar peas, fava beans, green beans; legumes including dried beans, lentils, chickpeas, lima beans, and soy beans).

Herbs and spices: tarragon, fenugreek seeds, nutmeg, licorice, senna, red clover.

Fruit: peaches, plums, apricots, cherries, nectarines, prunes, cape gooseberries, dates, grapes, raisins.

Oils, etc.: sunflower, safflower, soy and almond oils (tropical oils—coconut or palm oil if available), wine vinegar, Balsamic vinegar.

Suggested menus

Breakfasts

Fresh fruit salad

Compote of apricots and peaches

Rice porridge with prunes or Hunza apricots (p.83)

Rice pancakes with apricot or plum purée (p.87)

Rice flake muesli (p.84)

Soups and starters

Spinach and egg drop soup (p.110)

Green pea soup (p.110)

Bean sprouts and noodle soup (p.108)

Stuffed vine leaves (p.115)

Spinach and tofu puffs (p.121)

Almond- and date-stuffed peaches (p.120)

Chicken liver pâté (p.112)

Main meal dishes

Turkey and apricot pilaf (p.127)

Stir-fry duck with snow peas (p.127)

Pot roast pheasant/wild game bird (p.133)

Chicken with beets (p.126)

Roast chicken with plum stuffing (p.124)

Pigeon with prunes (p.132)

Vegetarian main meals

Artichoke and three-bean casserole (p.182)

Spinach and lentil flan (p.172)

Tempeh or tofu stir-fry (p.166)

Aduki bean burgers (p.163)

Spinach roulade with chickpea and salsify filling (p.183)

Apricot and almond pilaff (p.166)

Vegetables and salads

Cherry and almond salad (p.207)

Green bean salad (p.205)

Roasted Jerusalem artichokes (p.188)

Egg/tofu mayonnaise (p.195)

Puddings and desserts

Damson syllabub (p.227)

Chicory coffee ice cream (p.225)

Apricot and almond flan (p.228)

Cakes and biscuits

Sticky prune cake (p.216)

Rich fruit cake (p.215)

Carob and coconut brownies (p.217)

Cherry and coconut slices (p.221)

Rice bread (p.209)

Raisin bun loaf (p.209)

Drinks and miscellaneous

Rice milk (p.234)

Hot chocolate (p.235)

Soy milk (p.236)

Honey eggnog (p.236)

Almond and sunflower seed butters (p.238)

Day 4

The following foods can be eaten:

Cereals: buckwheat, buckwheat flour, buckwheat flakes and buckwheat pasta, sweet potato flour, chestnut flour, tapioca, amaranth, amaranth flour, and amaranth pasta.

Meat, etc.: beef, lamb, sheep's milk product, goat's milk products, cheese, butter, ghee, saltwater fish (cod, tuna, mackerel, eel, halibut, flounder, anchovy, sole, sardine, hake, haddock).

Nuts & seeds: hazelnuts and spread, walnuts, pecan nuts, chestnuts, poppy seeds, mustard seeds.

Sugars: maple syrup, apple and pear concentrate.

Drinks: sheep's milk, goat's milk, coffee, apple/pear juice, raspberry juice, raspberry leaf tea, rose-hip tea, Equisetum tea, lemongrass tea.

Vegetables: the mustard family (bok choy, cabbage, watercress, salad mustard and cress, mustard seed, cauliflower, broccoli, turnip, radish, horseradish, sprouts, kale, kohlrabi, rutabaga); sweet potatoes; yams; dasheen, eddoes; sorrel.

Herbs and spices: the myrtle family (cloves, allspice), mustard seeds, lemongrass, capers.

Fruit: pear, apple, loquat, quince, lychees, the rose family (strawberries, raspberries, blackberries, rose-hip), pectin, rhubarb, guava.

Oils, etc.: hazelnut oil, walnut oil, cider vinegar, raspberry vinegar.

Suggested menus

Breakfasts

Buckwheat and amaranth porridge (p.83)

Buckwheat muesli (p.85)

Amaranth and apple pancakes (p.88)

Compote of strawberries and rhubarb

Soups and starters

Turnip and watercress soup (p.94)

Kohlrabi and goat's cheese soup (p.107)

Oxtail soup (p.109)

Pears with stilton (p.122)

Tuna fish roll (p.123)

Sprout and chestnut dip (p.117)

Lamb's liver with raspberries (p.120)

Main meal dishes

Fillet of beef with caper sauce (p.142)

Pot roast brisket of beef with horseradish sauce (p.143)

Lamb burgers (p.136)

Buckwheat and walnut coated herrings (p.155)

Grilled halibut with anchovy butter (p.155)

Fisherman's pie (p.154)

Vegetarian main meals

Feta cheese and cabbage pie (p.173)

Buckwheat pasta with broccoli and walnuts (p.176)

Buckwheat chapatis (p.212)

Vegetables and salads

Horseradish sauce (p.197)

Mustard sauce (p.194)

Fresh green salad (p.198)

Fresh winter salad (p.198)

Pear and watercress salad (p.207)

Baked red cabbage (p.190)

Bubble and squeak nests (p.192)

Puddings and desserts

Tapioca milk pudding (p.227)

Steamed apple pudding (p.229)

Bramble mousse (p.229)

Pears in raspberry sauce (p.230)

Cakes and biscuits

Buckwheat and chestnut dropped scones (p.220)

Apple and hazelnut muffins (p.219)

Drinks and miscellaneous

Strawberry yogurt crush (p.232)

Rose hip cordial (p.232)

Hazelnut, walnut, or pecan nut butter (p.239)

chapter 6
the recipes

BREAKFAST

Quinoa porridge

Good for: Preliminary Diet; Elimination Diet, Days 6, 8 &10;
Rotation Diet, Day 3

Serves 1

¾ cup quinoa (preferably soaked overnight)

2 cups mineral water

Place the quinoa in a saucepan and add the mineral water. Bring
to a boil and simmer for 20 to 30 minutes, or until well cooked.
Millet porridge (see page 39) can be made in the same way,
replacing the quinoa with millet.

Speedy oat porridge

Good for: Rotation Diet, Day 2

Serves 2

1 cup organic rolled oats

4¼ cups water

Place the oats in a saucepan and add the cold water. Bring to a boil
and simmer for 1 minute, stirring as it thickens.

Sorghum porridge

Good for: Elimination Diet, Day 8; Rotation Diet, Day 2

Serves 2

⅔ cup sorghum meal

4¼ cups water

pinch of salt

Cook like the speedy oat porridge, stirring all the time.

Millet and kamut porridge

Good for: Elimination Diet, Day 11; Rotation Diet, Day 1

Serves 2

¾ cup millet flakes

¼ cup kamut, soaked overnight

2 cups water

Place the grains and flakes in a saucepan and add the water. Bring to a boil and simmer for 4 to 5 minutes until the kamut is soft and the porridge thickens. Serve with barley malt, chopped figs, or cashew nut milk.

Old-fashioned oatmeal porridge

Good for: Elimination Diet, Day 16; Rotation Diet, Day 2

Serves 2 to 3

1 cup pinhead oatmeal or whole oat groats

4¼ cups water

pinch of salt

Place the oats in a saucepan (double boiler if available), add the cold water and salt and bring to a boil. Turn off the heat and leave overnight. The next morning, bring to a boil again and simmer for 30 minutes, stirring from time to time.

Buckwheat and amaranth porridge

Good for: Rotation Diet, Day 4

Serves 2 to 3

⅓ cup amaranth, soaked overnight

1¾ cups buckwheat flakes

4¼ cups water

pinch of sea salt

Place the grains and flakes in a saucepan and add the water and salt. Bring to a boil and simmer gently for about 5 minutes until the amaranth is soft and the porridge thickens, stirring occasionally.

Rice porridge with prunes or hunza apricots

Good for: Elimination Diet, Day 12; Rotation Diet, Day 3

Serves 4

1 cup organic short wholegrain rice

8½ cups water

prunes or dried hunza apricots

Bring all the ingredients to a boil, then simmer very gently for a good hour until all the water has been absorbed. Cooking the rice in this way helps to preserve the nutrients and makes a very digestible and cleansing food for the gut.

Hunza apricots are the best, and are available at some health-food stores or may be ordered. Soak overnight and then cook for 7 to 10 minutes. Once soaked, the hunza apricots may also be eaten uncooked. The kernels can be cracked open and eaten as nuts. Prepare prunes in the same way as the apricots. Buy prunes and apricots from health-food stores and avoid the "ready-to-eat, no-need-to-soak" preparations.

Barley flake muesli

Good for: Rotation Diet, Day 1

Serves 4

2 cups barley flakes or a mixture of flakes from wheat, rye, or millet grains

cashew nuts

ground linseeds

sesame seeds

chopped dried or fresh figs

mango

Mix together all the ingredients and serve with mango or orange juice or cashew nut milk.

Rice flake muesli

Good for: Preliminary Diet; Rotation Diet, Day 3

Serves 4

rice flakes

chopped nuts

dried fruit or top with fresh fruit

soy, rice, or nut milks

Soak the rice flakes in liquid for 5 to 10 minutes before serving. Mix together all the ingredients and serve with mango or orange juice, cashew nut milk, grape juice, or the juice left over from cooking prunes and apricots.

Oat flake muesli

Good for: Rotation Diet, Day 2

Serves 4

2⅔ cups jumbo oatflakes

½ cup oat bran and germ (optional)

chopped Brazil nuts

pumpkin seeds

fresh or sundried bananas

Mix together all the ingredients and serve with pineapple juice, stewed gooseberries, or tiger nut milk.

Buckwheat muesli

Good for: Elimination Diet, Days 7 & 15; Rotation Diet, Day 4

Serves 4

2 cups buckwheat flakes

⅓ cup flaked or whole hazelnuts

⅓ cup pecan nut pieces

fresh or dried fruit, e.g., apples, pears, raspberries, chopped

sheep's milk, rice milk, or permitted fruit juice

rice syrup or maple syrup (optional)

Mix together all the dry ingredients and leave to soak with the milk or fruit juice for 5 to 7 minutes to soften. If you choose, serve with rice syrup or maple syrup.

Polenta (corn meal)

Good for: Elimination Diet, Day 16; Rotation Diet, Day 2

Serves 4

2½ cups water

1 tsp sea salt

1½ cups fine corn meal (polenta)

In a heavy-based saucepan, bring the water to a boil with the salt, and gradually add the corn meal, stirring with a wooden spoon to keep it smooth. Cook gently for 20 minutes until it thickens and comes cleanly away from the sides of the pan.

Pour into a well-oiled, shallow baking dish, approximately 8" x 12". Spread out with a wet spatula so the polenta is roughly ¼" thick.

Frumenty

Good for: Rotation Diet, Day 1

Serves 4

2½ cups organic whole wheat grains

4¼ cups water

Wash the wheat grains and presoak for 6 to 8 hours. Place in a pan with the remaining water and bring to a boil. Simmer gently for 10 minutes and then leave in a warm place overnight.

At the end of this time, the wheat grains should have burst open and look starchy and white and form a thick jelly. If some are still whole, boil up again and cook gently for a little while longer. Serve with fruit for breakfast or supper.

SOUPS AND STARTERS

Vegetable stock (potassium broth)

Good for: Preliminary Diet

Serves 4

Use vegetables, seaweeds, and trimmings but note that too many mustard family greens or spinach may spoil the flavor. Simmer gently, with plenty of water and with the lid on the saucepan for 1½ to 2 hours. The nutrients will leach into the stock, which can then be strained off and the fiber remains discarded. Take great care to label containers with all the ingredients, particularly if you are freezing the stock and when checking your allergies.

Lamb stock

Good for: Preliminary Diet

Serves 4

Use raw bones from organically reared mutton or lamb, chopped into 2" pieces. Wash and place in a large, heavy saucepan or pressure cooker. Cover with cold water and a pinch of salt and bring to a boil. Simmer for 3 hours or for 1½ hours in a pressure cooker. Strain the stock and allow to cool. Skim off the fat before use.

The stock may be frozen in an ice-cube tray or kept in a refrigerator for up to 2 days.

Poultry or game stock

Good for: Rotation Diet, Day 3

Serves 4

Turkey, duck, goose, chicken, or game stock can be made from the carcass, giblets, skin, and legs of the bird. Cook for 1½ hours (45 minutes in a pressure cooker), strain, allow to cool, and skim off the fat.

Fish stock

Good for: Preliminary Diet

Serves 4

Wash the trimmings and break up the bones. Cover with cold water, add a little sea salt, and bring to simmering point. Cook gently for no longer than 30 minutes to avoid bitterness. Use or freeze.

Cream of cauliflower soup with almonds

Good for: Preliminary Diet; Rotation Diet, Day 3

Serves 4

4¼ cups mineral water or stock

1 small sweet potato, peeled and roughly chopped

1 small cauliflower

3 ribs celery

sea salt

¾ cup ground almonds

Bring the water to a boil. Add the sweet potato, cauliflower, and celery and a pinch of salt. Cook for 5 to 7 minutes until the vegetables are tender.

Allow to cool slightly. Take out a few cauliflower florets. Add the ground almonds and blend until smooth. Return to the pan. Add the cauliflower florets and reheat gently.

Celery and zucchini soup

Good for: Preliminary Diet

Serves 4

4¼ cups stock or mineral water

6 ribs celery, diced

2 zucchini, cut lengthways and sliced

1 small sweet potato or yam, diced

sea salt or kelp

fresh cilantro, chopped

Bring the stock/water to a boil and add the vegetables and season. Cover and cook for 10 minutes until the vegetables are tender. Ladle out half the vegetables and blend to a purée. Return to the pan, reheat, and serve with a garnishing of cilantro or other fresh herb.

Celery and chestnut soup

Good for: Preliminary Diet

Serves 4

1 cup dried chestnuts, soaked

4¼ cups stock or mineral water

1 bunch of celery, roughly sliced

1 bay leaf

sea salt

freshly chopped parsley

Cook the chestnuts in half the water for 1 hour. Meanwhile, steam the celery or gently sauté in olive oil, reserving 1 or 2 finely diced stalks for garnishing. Cool slightly and blend to a purée with the chestnuts. Add the remaining stock or water and bay leaf and some salt. Reheat and serve with the diced celery and parsley.

Green split pea soup with broccoli

Good for: Preliminary Diet

Serves 4

1 cup green split peas

4¼ cups stock and/or mineral water

2 bay leaves

½ tsp dried marjoram

½ tsp lemongrass

1 tsp salt

2½ cups broccoli, chopped

¾ cup broccoli florets

Presoak the split peas in hot water for 1 to 2 hours (they will not sprout). Place in a pan with the water, bay leaves, herbs, and seasoning and cook for about 30 minutes until tender. Add the chopped broccoli and any remaining stock and cook for another 10 minutes. Remove the bay leaves and leave to cool slightly. Blend until smooth, and return to the pan to reheat.

Meanwhile, steam the broccoli florets in a little water until tender but still green, and add to the soup.

Turnip and watercress soup

Good for: Elimination Diet, Day 5; can be adapted for Rotation Day 4 by adding yogurt or cheese

Serves 4

1 bunch watercress

4¼ cups lamb stock and/or mineral water

3 cups turnips, peeled and roughly chopped

sea salt

Wash the watercress and separate the stalks from the leaves. Bring the stock/water to a boil and add the turnips. Simmer until tender. Blend with the watercress stalks and return to the pan. Add seasoning and the sprigs of watercress and cook another minute.

Cream of carrot and celery soup

Good for: Preliminary Diet; Elimination Diet, Day 7

Serves 4

1¾ cups carrots, chopped

1¾ cups celery, chopped

4¼ cups mineral water, game stock, or parsley family stock

sea salt

2½ tbsp olive oil

2½ tbsp chopped parsley or cilantro for garnishing

Cook the vegetables in some of the stock/water, until tender. Blend until smooth and creamy. Return to the pan, add seasoning and the remaining liquid, and reheat. Cook for another 2 minutes, add the oil, and serve with a garnishing of chopped parsley.

Yam and Belgian endive soup

Good for: Elimination Diet, Day 8

Serves 4

1 cup mineral water/stock

1½ cups yam, peeled and chopped

sea salt

2 heads of Belgin endive, chopped

1 tbsp fresh tarragon, chopped, for garnishing

Bring the water to a boil. Add the yam and a pinch of salt. Bring to a boil and simmer until tender. Blend and return to the pan. Add the endive and cook for 1 minute. Sprinkle with tarragon and serve.

Swiss chard and celery soup

Good for: Elimination Diet, Day 10

Serves 4

4 sticks celery
4½ cups Swiss chard or spinach
1 cup sweet potato or yam
4¼ cups stock or water
sea salt
fresh thyme or ½ tsp dried

Reserve a celery stick and a leaf of Swiss chard. Roughly chop the remaining vegetables and boil in a little water, in order of cooking time. Blend in a blender and return to the saucepan with the stock/water and bring to a boil. Season with salt and thyme and add the reserved leaf of Swiss chard cut into slivers and the celery stick thinly sliced. Cook for another 2 minutes.

Onion and barley soup

Good for: Elimination Diet, Day 15

Serves 4

3 cups onions thinly sliced
1 cup pot barley
1 bay leaf
4¼ cups game or vegetable stock or water
arame seaweed, washed and soaked
olive oil
1 tbsp tamari soy sauce
chopped parsley for garnishing

Place the onions, barley, and bay leaf in a pan and cover with half the water/stock. Cook for 20 minutes until the barley is soft. Add the arame seaweed and soaking water and the remaining stock and bring to boiling point. Simmer another 10 minutes. Stir in the olive oil and tamari sauce and garnish with chopped parsley.

the allergy exclusion diet

Cream of asparagus soup

Good for: Elimination Diet, Day 11

Serves 4

3⅔ cups asparagus

1 large onion

4¼ cups game or vegetable stock or water

⅓ cup ground almonds

sea salt

juice of 1 lemon

1 tbsp fresh parsley, chopped, for garnishing

Wash and prepare the asparagus. Cut off the tips and trim off the coarse outer parts of the remaining stems. Cut into ⅝" pieces. Cook the tips in a little water and drain, reserving the water. The tips are not needed in this recipe.

Cook the onion and the asparagus stems in the water for 5 to 7 minutes until soft. Make up the quantity of liquid with the stock/water and add the ground almonds and salt. Blend the soup to a creamy constituency and serve with chopped parsley. Serve with the lemon juice and a garnishing of chopped parsley.

Baked tomato soup

Good for: Elimination Diet, Day 12; Rotation Diet, Day 2

Serves 4

3⅔ cups tomatoes,

1 onion, sliced

2 cloves garlic

4¼ cups pork stock or water

2½ tbsp freshly chopped basil

sea salt

Preheat the oven to 350°F. Cut the tomatoes into halves and scoop out the seeds. Place on a baking tray with the onion and garlic cloves and bake for 20 minutes. Remove from the oven and take the skins off the tomatoes. Cool slightly and then blend.

Bring the stock/water to a boil and add the baked ingredients together with the basil and salt. Cook for 5 minutes and serve with a sprinkling of basil.

Miso soup

Good for: Elimination Diet, Day 16

Serves 4

1 carrot, diced

½ small cauliflower, broken into florets

⅓ cup peas

4 spring onions sliced

1 clove garlic, crushed

1 tsp grated ginger

4¼ cups water

1 tbsp miso soy bean paste

2 sheets nori seaweed cut into ¾" squares

Gently cook the vegetables and seasonings in the water until soft. Blend the miso in a little of the soup liquid and add to the soup but do not allow to boil. Add the nori and serve.

Yellow split pea soup

Good for: Elimination Diet, Day 13

Serves 4

1 cup yellow split peas, soaked

4¼ cups stock or water

1 tsp caraway seeds

1 bay leaf

sea salt

3 ribs celery, chopped

1¼ cup yams or sweet potatoes, diced

2½ tbsp olive oil

parsley, for garnishing

Allow the split peas to soak in hot water for 1 to 2 hours (these have been processed and will not sprout). Cook the peas, gently with the seasoning, for 40 minutes until beginning to turn mushy. Remove the bay leaf.

Cook the celery and potatoes in some of the water/stock until soft. Add to the split peas and blend until smooth. Return to the pan, add the remaining liquid, and reheat. Cook for 2 minutes. Stir in the olive oil and serve with a garnishing of chopped parsley.

Mushroom and black bean soup

Good for: Elimination Diet, Day 17

Serves 4

2 leeks, thinly sliced

4¼ cups stock or water

1¼ cups wild mushrooms, diced

2 cups black beans, soaked, sprouted and cooked

1 tbsp soy, gram, or barley flour

1 bay leaf

sprig of thyme

Cook the leeks until tender. Add the stock/water and bring to a boil. Mix in the mushrooms, beans, and seasoning and cook gently for 15 to 20 minutes. Remove the bay leaf and thyme and serve.

Leek and potato soup

Good for: Elimination Diet, Day 20

Serves 4

2½ cups potatoes, peeled and diced

3 leeks, sliced

2 bay leaves

sprig of rosemary

4¼ cups stock or water

sea salt

bunch of chives, chopped

creamed sheep's cheese or yogurt (optional)

Gently cook the vegetables, bay leaves, and rosemary in some of the stock/water for 20 minutes. Remove the rosemary and bay leaves. Allow to cool slightly and mix in a blender. Add the salt and chopped chives and reheat gently. May be served with sheep's cheese or yogurt.

Garden vegetable soup

Good for: Elimination Diet, Day 23

Serves 4

4¼ cups stock or water
1¼ cups small pickling onions
1 cup broccoli florets
2 carrots, thinly sliced
2 zucchini, diced
1 cup button mushrooms, quartered
1 tbsp barley or gram flour
sea salt or kelp
fresh thyme, for garnishing

Pour the stock/water into a saucepan and bring to a boil. Add all the ingredients, bring to a boil, and simmer until cooked.

Cream of artichoke soup

Good for: Elimination Diet, Day 24

Serves 4

4¼ cups chicken, game or vegetable stock
4½ cup Jerusalem artichokes, peeled and sliced
1 large onion, sliced
pinch of nutmeg
½ cup goat's milk yogurt
sprigs of watercress or freshly chopped tarragon for garnishing

Pour the stock into a saucepan and bring to a boil. Add the artichokes, onion, and seasoning and return to a boil. Cover and simmer for 20 minutes until all the vegetables are tender. Cool slightly and blend until smooth. Reheat and serve with goat's milk yogurt and a garnishing of watercress or tarragon.

Chicken noodle main meal soup

Good for: Elimination Diet, Day 27

Serves 4

2½ cups water or stock

8 ounces free-range chicken breast

¾ cup fresh peas

4 spring onions sliced

2 carrots, diced

1 tsp grated ginger

1 tsp ground cilantro (coriander)

½ tsp ground turmeric

sea salt or kelp

1 cup coconut milk

1¼ cups rice noodles

cilantro for garnishing

Pour the water/stock into a saucepan and bring to a boil. Cut the chicken into thin strips and add to the pan to seal. Add the vegetables and spices and bring to a boil. Cover and simmer for 35 minutes. Add the coconut milk and noodles and simmer, stirring for another 5 to 8 minutes. Garnish with chopped cilantro and serve.

Minestrone soup

Good for: Elimination Diet, Day 28

Serves 4

4¼ cups stock

1 potato, diced

2 carrots, cut in half lengthways and thinly sliced

2 bay leaves

2½ cups tomatoes, skinned and diced

¾ cup green beans, cut into short pieces

1 zucchini, diced

2 onions, chopped

2 cloves garlic, crushed

sea salt

½ cup white cabbage, shredded

2½ tbsp fresh basil or oregano, chopped

2 cups flageolet beans, sprouted and cooked

5 ounces wholemeal pasta shapes (wheat, barley, millet or rice), cooked

grated Parmesan cheese (optional)

Pour the stock into a pan, bring to a boil; and add the potato, carrots, bay leaves, and the remaining vegetables in order of cooking time and season. Simmer for 20 minutes and then add the shredded cabbage, basil, flageolet beans, and pasta and cook for another 2 to 3 minutes. Remove the bay leaves and serve with Parmesan cheese.

Avocado and green pepper soup

Good for: Rotation Diet, Day 2

Serves 4

2 green peppers, deseeded and chopped

4¼ cups stock or water

2 bay leaves

sea salt

2 large avocados

freshly chopped mint, for garnishing

Cook the peppers in a little of the stock/water with the bay leaves and a pinch of salt in a saucepan until tender. Remove the bay leaves.

Peel and remove pit of the avocado and place the flesh in a blender. Pour in the contents of the saucepan. Blend to a purée and return to the saucepan to reheat, adding the remaining stock. Serve with a sprinkling of chopped mint.

Spiced pumpkin and ginger soup

Good for: Elimination Diet, Day 22; Rotation Diet, Day 2

Serves 4

5 cups pumpkin or squash flesh, diced

1 tsp root ginger, grated

2 cloves garlic, crushed

1 dried chilli, crushed

1 tsp ground turmeric

sea salt

4¼ cups stock or water

Place all the ingredients in a large saucepan. Cover with some of the water/stock and bring to a boil. Simmer for 10 minutes and allow to cool slightly. Place in a blender and mix until smooth. Return to the saucepan, adding the remaining stock, and cook for another 5 minutes.

Parsnip and cilantro soup

Good for: Rotation Diet, Day 1

Serves 4

4¼ cups vegetable stock

4½ cups parsnips, diced

2 ribs celery, sliced

sea salt or kelp

½ tsp ground coriander

½ tsp ground cumin

2½ tbsp fresh cilantro, chopped, for garnishing

Place half the stock in a saucepan and bring to a boil. Add the parsnips, celery, salt or kelp and ground spices and cook until tender. Cool slightly and then blend to a purée. Return to the pan with the remaining stock and reheat. Serve with a garnishing of fresh cilantro.

Mushroom and barley broth

Good for: Rotation Diet, Day 1

Serves 4

2¼ cups mushrooms, diced

1¾ cups pot barley

2 carrots, diced

4¼ cups stock or water

sea salt or 1¼ tsp barley miso

2 tbsp chopped parsley for garnishing

Put all the ingredients into a casserole dish, bring to a boil, cover with a lid, and simmer gently for 40 to 50 minutes until the barley is cooked, adding more liquid if necessary. Serve with a sprinkling of chopped parsley.

Clear vegetable and nori broth

Good for: Rotation Diet, Day 1

Serves 4

4¼ cups vegetable, lamb, or fish stock or water

2 large carrots, cut into matchsticks

2 ribs celery, thinly sliced

1 small parsnip, diced

1 tsp barley miso, sea salt, kelp

2 to 3 sheets nori seaweed, cut into ¾" squares

1 tbsp sesame seed oil

Place some of the water/stock in a pan and bring to a boil. Add the vegetables and cook until tender. Add the remaining stock, miso, and nori seaweed, bring to a boil, and simmer for 1 minute. Stir in the sesame seed oil and serve.

Fish and fennel soup

Good for: Rotation Diet, Day 1

Serves 4

4¼ cups fish or vegetable stock or water

1 head of fennel, cut into strips

2 carrots, diced

1 tsp dried fennel

sea salt or 1 tsp kelp

5 ounces freshwater fish, filleted

5 ounces mixed shellfish, shelled

2 ounces small pasta shells

2 tbsp fresh parsley, chopped

Bring some of the stock/water to a boil and cook the fennel and carrots until just tender. Add the remaining liquid, dried fennel, and salt or kelp, and re-boil. Add the fish and pasta and cook for another 5 minutes, adding the parsley during the last minute of cooking. Cook the pasta separately if a larger, longer cooking variety is used.

Kohlrabi and goat's cheese soup

Good for: Rotation Diet, Day 4

Serves 4

3 cups kohlrabi, diced

1 small sweet potato, diced

4¼ cups stock or water

½ cup soft goat's cheese

½ tsp allspice

sea salt

watercress, for garnishing

Cook the kohlrabi and sweet potato in the stock/water until tender. Remove the rind from the goat's cheese and blend with the vegetables. Add the seasoning and reheat. Serve with a sprinkling of chopped watercress.

Sweetcorn and lima bean succotash soup

Good for: Elimination Diet, Day 18

Serves 4

¾ cup yam, diced

¾ cup zucchini, diced

2 ribs celery, sliced

1 cup vegetable stock or water

2⅓ cups lima beans, sprouted and cooked

2 cups sweetcorn kernels

1 sprig thyme

3 sage leaves, chopped

2 tbsp olive oil

sea salt

Cook the yam, zucchini, and celery in the stock/water for 5 to 7 minutes in order of cooking time. Add the remaining ingredients and simmer for 10 minutes.

Lentil soup

Good for: Preliminary Diet; Elimination Diet, Day 9

Serves 4

4¼ cups water or stock

1⅔ cups brown lentils, presoaked

2 large carrots, roughly chopped

1 parsnip, roughly chopped

2 ribs celery, roughly chopped

1 tsp cumin seeds

sea salt

1 tbsp chopped cilantro, for garnishing

Bring the water/stock to a boil. Add the lentils, vegetables, cumin seeds, and salt. Simmer gently until the vegetables are tender. Blend and return to the pan to reheat. Serve with a sprinkling of fresh cilantro.

Bean sprouts and noodle soup

Good for: Rotation Diet, Day 3

Serves 4

1½ cups chickpea sprouts

1½ cups lentil sprouts

1½ cups mung bean sprouts

4¼ cups water

3 stalks Swiss chard, sliced

1 to 2 tsp miso or sea salt

2 ounces rice noodles

Chop the chickpeas and place in a large saucepan together with the lentil and mung bean sprouts and cover with boiling water. Cook for 10 to 15 minutes until tender. Add the Swiss chard, miso or salt, and rice noodles, and cook another 7 to 10 minutes.

Gazpacho

Good for: Rotation Diet, Day 2

Serves 4

2¼ cups tomatoes peeled, deseeded and chopped

1 cup stock or water

¼ cup olive oil

2 onions, chopped

1 large cucumber, peeled and diced

1 large green pepper, deseeded and diced

2 cloves garlic, crushed

black pepper

Blend half the tomatoes, stock, and olive oil into a purée. Mix in with the vegetables and refrigerate for 2 to 4 hours before serving.

Oxtail soup

Good for: Rotation Diet, Day 4

Serves 4

2 small oxtails from organically reared beef

4¼ cups water

2 small turnips, halved and sliced

¾ cup rutabaga, diced

1 tsp mustard seeds

sea salt

1 tbsp tapioca flour

Wash and dry the oxtails and cut into joints. Put the water in a saucepan and bring to a boil. Add the oxtail joints, vegetables, and seasoning, and return to a boil. Simmer gently for 3 hours or pressure cook for 1½ hours. Take out the pieces of oxtail and cut the meat from the bone. Return the meat to the soup and reheat. Mix the tapioca flour with a little cold water and stir into the soup.

There may be some fat on the soup, which can be removed with a baster or allow to cool overnight and skim the fat from the top.

Green pea soup

Good for: Rotation Diet, Day 3

Serves 4

3 cups fresh peas in their pods
1 head of romaine lettuce
4¼ cups water
sea salt
½ cup soy cream

Shell the peas and reserve the pods. Take the outer leaves from the lettuce and cook with the pods for 10 minutes in some of the water. Cool a little and blend to a purée. Pour through a sieve and discard the pulp.

Place the stock to one side and bring the remaining water to a boil. Add the peas, sliced lettuce leaves, and salt, and cook for 7 to 10 minutes. Blend and return to the pan with the pea stock. Reheat and stir in the soy cream, if using, before serving.

This soup may also be served with shredded smoked tofu instead of soy cream.

Spinach and eggdrop soup

Good for: Rotation Diet, Day 3

Serves 4

3 cups spinach, washed and chopped
4¼ cups chicken stock or water
½ tsp nutmeg
2 tsp miso or sea salt
2 eggs, lightly beaten

Place the spinach in a saucepan and cover with boiling stock/water. Cook for 3 to 4 minutes until tender. Cool slightly, then blend to a purée. Return to the pan, add the remaining stock/water, nutmeg, and seasoning and reheat. Remove from the heat and add the eggs, stirring until they separate into strands. Serve immediately.

Pistachio and rabbit pâté

Good for: Rotation Diet, Day 1

Serves 4

1 tbsp sesame seed oil

1 lb boneless rabbit meat and/or rabbit livers

1⅔ cups celery root, diced

1 cup water or stock

2 tbsp chopped parsley

1 rounded tbsp barley or wheat flour

¾ cup pistachio nuts, chopped

sea salt

black pepper

Warm the sesame seed oil and a little water in a pan and gently cook the rabbit meat on both sides for 4 to 5 minutes. Put to one side and cook the celery root in the juices until soft. Add the water/stock and parsley and bring to a boil. Simmer for 2 to 3 minutes. Mix the flour with a little cold water and stir into the liquid to make a thick sauce. Cool slightly and blend with the meat to make a smooth paste. Turn into a bowl and stir in the pistachio nuts, salt, and pepper and serve chilled with bread or crackers.

Chicken liver pâté

Good for: Rotation Diet, Day 3

Serves 4

FOR THE WHITE SAUCE

1 rounded tbsp rice flour

1 cup soy/nut milk or stock (or a mixture)

FOR THE PÂTÉ

4 chicken livers

1 tbsp dripping

1 cup thick white sauce

1 egg

1 tbsp freshly chopped tarragon

pinch of nutmeg

sea salt

To make the white sauce, mix the rice flour with a little water. Bring the milk/stock to a boil and stir in the rice flour. Cook until the sauce thickens.

For the pâté, wash and trim the livers. Heat the dripping in a pan and cook the livers gently until just cooked. Cool slightly and place in a food processor with the white sauce and the remaining ingredients. Blend until smooth and turn into a pâté dish and refrigerate.

Avocado and zucchini dip

Good for: Rotation Diet, Day 2

Serves 4

2 large ripe avocados

¾ cup cooked zucchini

2 cloves garlic, crushed

sea salt

paprika pepper

FOR THE CRUDITÉS

1 red, yellow, and green pepper, deseeded and cut lengthways

1 cucumber, cut into 2" chunks and then cut lengthways

baby corn

Scoop out the flesh of the avocados and mash together with the cooked zucchini. Add the seasoning and serve with crudités or tortillas.

Sprout and chestnut dip

Good for: Rotation Diet, Day 4

Serves 4

2¼ cups Brussels sprouts

1½ cups cooked chestnuts

1 tsp ground lemongrass

sea salt

FOR THE CRUDITÉS

raw rutabaga, cut into pieces

turnip or kohlrabi, cut into matchsticks

radishes, cauliflower florets, bok choy

Cook the Brussels sprouts in a little water for 3 to 4 minutes until soft. Cool slightly and blend with the chestnuts and seasoning. Blend to a smooth purée adding some of the cooking water if necessary. Allow to cool and serve with the crudités.

Hummus and cannellini bean dip

Good for: Elimination Diet, Day 16

Serves 4

3 cups chickpeas, sprouted and cooked; or 3 cups cannellini beans, sprouted

¼ cup tahini

juice of 2 lemons

2 cloves garlic

1½ tbsp olive oil

1 tbsp sesame seed oil

black pepper, sea salt

parsley and paprika pepper, or fresh mint and ground cumin for garnishing

For the hummus, place the chickpeas and all the remaining ingredients in a food processor and mix until smooth using some of the chickpea cooking water if necessary. Serve with crudités—sticks of carrot, celery, green, red and yellow peppers, cauliflower florets, radishes, Belgian endive, etc.

For the cannellini bean dip, follow the recipe for hummus using sprouted cannellini beans instead of chickpeas, and flavor with chopped fresh mint and ground cumin. Garnish with a sprig of mint.

Tomato relish

Good for: Elimination Diet, Day 28

Serves 4

1¼ cups tomatoes, skinned, seeded, and chopped

4 spring onions, chopped

¼ cup capers

1 stick celery, chopped

paprika pepper

1 tbsp tomato purée

freshly chopped basil

pinch of allspice

sea salt

Mix together the ingredients and use as required.

Sweetcorn relish

Good for: Elimination Diet, Day 28

Serves 4

1⅓ cups sweetcorn

1 red pepper, deseeded and chopped

½ cucumber, diced

½ tsp chili powder (optional)

½ tsp ground mustard

black pepper

sea salt

Place half the sweetcorn in a blender and mix. Combine with the remaining ingredients.

Date and apple chutney

Good for: Elimination Diet, Day 28

Serves 4

1 cup cider vinegar

2¼ cups eating apples, chopped

2¼ cups cooking apples, chopped

1⅓ cups pitted dates, chopped

1½ cups golden raisins

1½ cups onions, chopped

⅔ cup raw cane molasses sugar (optional)

1 tsp grated ginger

pinch of allspice

sea salt

Bring the vinegar to a boil and add all the ingredients. Cook for 15 to 20 minutes until tender and the cooking apples have become mushy. Keep refrigerated, or it may be bottled or frozen.

Lamb's liver with raspberries

Good for: Rotation Diet, Day 4

Serves 4

1¾ cups raspberries

2½ tsp maple syrup

2½ tbsp raspberry vinegar

8 ounces lamb's liver

sea salt

bok choy for garnishing

Reserve 12 raspberries for garnishing, and purée the remainder in a blender. Strain and stir in the maple syrup and vinegar.

Cut the liver into thin strips, sprinkle with a little salt, and grill for 3 to 4 minutes, turning until all sides are cooked. Arrange the liver on four warmed plates and pour over the raspberry sauce. Garnish with Chinese leaves.

Almond- and date-stuffed peaches

Good for: Rotation Diet, Day 3

Serves 4

2 large white peaches, peeled and halved

sea salt

1 small head of iceberg lettuce, shredded

½ cup silken tofu

¾ cup chopped dates

¾ cup almonds, cut into halves lengthways

alfalfa sprouts for garnishing

Rinse the peach halves in salted water to prevent browning, and remove the pits. Place on a bed of lettuce on individual plates. Cream the tofu and put a spoonful in the center of each peach. Arrange the dates and almonds on top with a few shreds of lettuce, and garnish with a sprinkling of alfalfa sprouts.

Spinach and tofu puffs

Good for: Rotation Diet, Day 3

Serves 4

FOR THE CHOUX PASTRY

¼ cup sunflower seed oil or safflower oil

½ tsp sea salt

½ cup water

1 cup rice flour

2 eggs

FOR THE FILLING

3⅔ cups spinach

1¼ cups silken tofu

2 tsp umeboshi purée or pinch of nutmeg and sea salt

Preheat the oven to 345°F.

For the choux pastry, place the oil, salt, and water in a pan and bring to a boil. Add the rice flour, beating with a wooden spoon to form a smooth dough. Allow to cool slightly, and gradually beat in the eggs to form a paste. Using two spoons or an icing bag with a ⅝" diameter nozzle, drop eight mounds of dough on a baking sheet, leaving room for the dough to expand. Bake for 20 to 25 minutes until the mounds are firm and golden. Using a serrated knife, slice the top off each puff and leave to cool.

For the filling, wash and drain the spinach and cook it in its own juices for 2 to 3 minutes until tender. Drain thoroughly and chop. Mix with the silken tofu and flavorings and beat to form a smooth paste. Spoon the mixture into the choux puffs and replace the tops. Serve hot or cold.

This recipe may also be made up as a choux ring. Pipe the pastry on to the baking tray to form a 8" diameter ring leaving 4" clear in the center.

Pears with stilton

Good for: Rotation Diet, Day 4

Serves 4

½ cup crème fraîche
¼ cup milk
½ cup Stilton cheese
1 tsp poppy seeds
2 large pears

Place the crème fraîche and milk in a saucepan over a gentle heat.
Crumble in the Stilton and stir until melted. Remove from the heat and
mix in the poppyseeds and divide between four small serving plates.

Cut the pears in half lengthways and remove the cores. Cut each
half into about eight segments, keeping the stalk end intact if
possible, and dip in and out of salt water to prevent browning.
Arrange in a fan shape on top of the cheese sauce.

Open sandwiches

Good for: Elimination Diet, Day 18

Spread slices of rye/pumpernickel rye bread with tahini, hummus, or
nut spread, and then add any of the following:

Fish salad: 1 sardine, 2 tomato wedges, lettuce leaf, cress, and lemon
slice.

Grape and tofu: slices of tofu, lettuce, tomato wedge, and 1 or 2
black grapes, halved and deseeded.

Sprouted bean salad: alfalfa sprouts, cucumber slices, and tomato
wedge.

Game bird: breast of pheasant, watercress, and slice of fresh orange.

Egg and tomato: slices of hard-boiled quail's eggs, 3 slices tomato,
lettuce, and parsley.

Prawn and salad: 2 ounces prawns, lettuce, 2 tomato wedges, lemon
wedge, and parsley.

Crab meal and salad: 2 ounces crabmeat, lettuce, 2 walnut halves,
watercress, and black olive.

Turkey and apricot pilaf

Good for: Elimination Diet, Day 8; Rotation Diet, Day 3

Serves 4

1.5 lbs turkey filet

1 cup stock or water

sea salt

½ tsp nutmeg

1 cup dried unsulphured apricots, pre-soaked

⅓ cup seedless golden raisins

1 cup whole-meal basmati rice

Divide the turkey fillets into smaller pieces as required. Place in a saucepan and cover with stock/water (you may use the soaking water from the apricots). Add the salt, nutmeg, and fruit, and cook for 20 minutes until the chicken is cooked through.

Meanwhile, cook the rice in 2 cups salted water for about 15 minutes until almost tender. Mix with the turkey and fruit, and cook for another 10 minutes until the rice is tender and has absorbed some of the juices.

Stir-fry duck with snow peas

Good for: Rotation Diet, Day 3

Serves 4

1 lb duckling breasts, cut into thin strips

2¼ cups snow peas, topped and tailed

2 cups bean sprouts

2 heads Belgian endive, sliced

2 tsps honey

1 tbsp Tamari soy sauce

⅓ cup almonds, cut lengthways, for garnishing

Heat a little water in a wok and add the strips of duck. Cook for 5 minutes and then add the snow peas, bean sprouts, and endive. Cook for another 7 to 10 minutes. Stir in the honey and soy sauce and garnish with almonds. Serve with brown rice.

Wild duck with pineapple

Good for: Preliminary Diet; Elimination Diet, Day 27

Serves 4

2 lb oven-ready wild duck

1 carrot, cut into strips

1 celery rib, sliced

1 cup stock or mineral water

1 bay leaf

1 sprig thyme

sea salt

1 small pineapple

Preheat the oven to 375°F.

Place the duck in an ovenproof casserole dish and add the vegetables, stock/water, bay leaf, thyme, and salt and cook for 1½ hours, reducing the oven temperature to 325°F after the first 15 minutes. Baste from time to time and add more water if necessary. When cooked, lift onto a serving dish.

Prepare the pineapple by removing the skin and cutting into slices ¼" thick and cook in the remaining juice, simmering for approximately 2 minutes. Remove the bay leaf and thyme. Garnish the duck with pineapple and pour over the juice.

Roast duck with orange and grapefruit sauce

Good for: Preliminary Diet; Elimination Diet, Day 19

Serves 4

4 lb oven-ready duck

2 small grapefruits

2 bay leaves

3 oranges

1 tsp corn starch or tapioca flour

2½ tbsp honey

Preheat the oven to 375°F.

Prick the duck all over with a fork. Sprinkle with salt and place half a grapefruit and 2 bay leaves in the body cavity.

Place on a rack or trivet, breast side down, in a roasting pan, and roast in the oven for 30 minutes. Reduce the oven temperature to 325°F and cook for another 1½ hours. Baste from time to time, and you can also, if you wish, remove the pan from the oven and pour off the excess fat and use this for roasting potatoes.

To prepare the sauce, squeeze the juice from the remaining grapefruit half and the juice from 1 orange. Peel the other grapefruit and 2 oranges and cut the peel into thin strips. Bring some water to a boil and blanche the strips of peel for 2 to 3 minutes. Drain and put to one side. Cut the oranges into thin slices and divide the grapefruit into segments.

When the duck is cooked, pour off the cooking juices and place the duck on a serving dish and keep warm in the turned-off oven. Skim off the excess fat from the roasting pan and place over medium heat. Mix the corn starch to a smooth paste with a little cold water, and add to the juices in the pan. Add the orange and grapefruit juices, the strips of peel and the honey, and simmer, stirring for 2 to 3 minutes until the sauce thickens. Pour around the duck. Garnish with the orange slices arranged along the breast, and the grapefruit segments round the dish, and serve immediately.

Game bird casserole

Good for: Preliminary Diet; Elimination Diet, Day 7

Serves 4

A couple of grouse, partridge, or 3 pigeons

3 to 4 carrots

1 parsnip

2 ribs of celery, sliced

2 tsp chopped parsley

sea salt

2½ cups boiling mineral water

2 tsp tapioca flour

Preheat the oven to 375°F.

Place the game birds in an ovenproof casserole dish. Add the vegetables—left whole or cut where necessary—parsley, and salt and pour in a boiling water. Cook for 1½ hours, reducing the temperature of the oven to 325°F after the first 20 minutes.

Place the game birds and the vegetables on a hot serving dish. Skim off any fat and use the cooking juices to make a gravy, using a little tapioca flour mixed with some cold water to thicken.

Roast quail with spring onion rice and cranberry sauce

Good for: Elimination Diet, Day 11

Serves 4

6 to 8 oven-ready quail (allow 1 to 2 per person)

sea salt

FOR THE SPRING ONION RICE

1 cup spring onions

1⅓ cups long-grain rice (a little wild rice may be used)

2 bay leaves

3⅔ cups water

FOR THE SAUCE

2¼ cups cranberries

½ cup water

1 clove garlic (optional)

grated zest and juice of 1 orange (optional)

pinch of cinnamon

2½ tbsp maple syrup or to taste

Preheat the oven to 350°F.

Place the quails in a casserole dish and sprinkle with salt. Cover and cook for 30 minutes.

To cook the rice, cut the spring onions into ¼" lengths and add the rice, bay leaves, salt, and water. Bring to a boil, cover, and simmer for 20 to 25 minutes until cooked. Remove the bay leaves before serving.

To make the cranberry sauce, place all the ingredients in a pan except for the maple syrup, and simmer gently for 2 to 3 minutes until the cranberries are tender. Add maple syrup to taste.

Place the rice on a serving dish and arrange the quails on the top. Serve with cranberry sauce.

Pigeon with prunes

Good for: Rotation Diet, Day 3

Serves 4

8 pigeon breasts

2½ cups stock or water

2 cups cooked prunes

2 tsp fresh tarragon chopped

pinch of nutmeg

sea salt

2 tsp sago flour

Place the pigeon breasts in a flameproof casserole dish and add the stock/water mixed with a little prune juice, and the remaining ingredients, except for the sago flour. Cover with a lid and cook over a gentle heat for 20 minutes. Lift out the pigeon breasts and place on a serving dish.

Mix the sago flour with some cold water and stir into the cooking stock to make a sauce. Pour over the pigeon breasts and arrange the prunes around. Serve on a bed of rice with diced green beans and peas.

Pot roast pheasant/wild game bird

Good for: Rotation Diet, Day 3

Serves 4

1 pheasant

salt

nutmeg

This is an excellent way of cooking game birds when the age and tenderness of the meat is unknown. Some pheasants are fed on corn, and this may affect some people. The same goes for corn-fed poultry.

Preheat the oven to 375°F.

Place the pheasant in a heavy-based casserole dish. Add enough boiling water to half cover, and season with salt and nutmeg. Cover and cook for 1 to 1½ hours, reducing the temperature to 325°F after the first 15 minutes, until the meat is tender and is just beginning to fall away from the bone.

Rabbit/hare hot pot

Good for: Preliminary Diet; Rotation Diet, Day 1

Serves 4

2 lb rabbit/hare portions

1 parsnip, diced

4 carrots, sliced

3 ribs celery, sliced

½ cup pot barley (use rice for Preliminary Diet)

sea salt or kelp

4¼ cups boiling water

2 tbsp freshly chopped parsley, for garnishing

Arrange the rabbit or hare portions in a heavy-based saucepan. Add the vegetables, barley, and salt and pour over a boiling water. Bring to a boil and simmer gently for 1½ hours. Add the chopped parsley and serve.

Pot roast rabbit with mushroom and fennel stuffing

Good for: Rotation Diet, Day 1

Serves 4

FOR THE STUFFING

2½ cups breadcrumbs or millet flakes

1¼ cups mushrooms, chopped

grated zest and juice of 1 lemon

1 bulb fennel, chopped

3¾ tbsp fresh parsley, chopped

1 tsp chopped chervil, if available

sea salt

1 large rabbit, skinned

2½ cups stock or water

Preheat the oven to 350°F.

Mix together the ingredients for the stuffing, adding a little water if necessary. Stuff the body of the rabbit and bring the open sides together, securing with string or skewers. Place in a casserole dish, pour over the stock/water, and place the lid on the top. Cook in the oven for 15 minutes. Reduce the temperature to 325°F and cook for another 45 minutes. Allow the rabbit to sit for 10 minutes before carving.

Lamb noisettes

Good for: Elimination Diet, Day 28

Serves 4

FOR THE TOPPING

¼ cup rice flakes

1 large onion, chopped

sea salt

knob of butter

¼ cup stock

1 egg yolk

1 tbsp yogurt

8 lamb cutlets trimmed

grated cheese

FOR GARNISHING

1¼ cups mushrooms, chopped

pat of butter

sea salt

1 tbsp mixed herbs, e.g. tarragon, mint, parsley

Preheat the oven to 325°F.

To prepare the topping, place the rice, onion, salt and a pat of butter in a pan and pour over the stock. Bring to a boil and simmer for 35 minutes. Sift the rice mixture and add the egg yolk and yogurt to make a smooth purée.

Prepare the cutlets, and grill on one side only for about 5 minutes with the bones all running the same way. Cover the cooked side of each cutlet with the purée, shaping it on neatly. Sprinkle with grated cheese and arrange on a baking tray and cook in the oven for 20 minutes.

For the garnish, peel and trim the mushrooms. Chop the stalks and sauté in butter for about 1 minute, without allowing the butter to brown. Add seasoning and herbs. Fill into the hollow of the mushrooms and pour over a little melted butter. Put on to a tray and cook in the oven with the cutlets for 10 minutes.

Lamb burgers

Good for: Preliminary Diet; Rotation Diet, Day 4

Serves 4

6 oz lean lamb
2 oz lamb's liver
1 cup chestnut flour
sea salt

Mince the lamb and the liver. Mix together with the chestnut flour and seasoning and shape into 4 burgers about 1" thick, or use a burger press. Grill for 4 to 5 minutes on each side.

Vegetarian/lamb shepherd's pie

Good for: Elimination Diet, Day 28

Serves 4

2 onions, sliced
2 carrots, diced
1 ribs celery, diced
1 zucchini, diced
3 cups brown lentils, sprouted and cooked
1¼ cups buckwheat or pot barley, cooked
¾ cups hazelnuts, chopped
tamari or teriyaki soy sauce
2 cups potatoes, cooked and mashed
½ cup Cheddar cheese (optional)
Lentils, buckwheat, and hazelnuts may be replaced with 2½ cups of cooked, minced lamb.

Preheat the oven to 325°F.
    Steam or boil the vegetables until tender. Mix with the lentils, buckwheat, hazelnuts, and soy sauce and turn into a well-oiled oven-safe dish. Top with the mashed potato, sprinkle with cheese, if using, and bake for 30 to 35 minutes.

Pot roast leg of lamb

Good for: Elimination Diet, Day 26

Serves 4

4 lbs leg of lamb

sea salt

3 to 4 sprigs of rosemary

2 carrots, sliced

1 parsnip, sliced lengthways

2 ribs of celery, sliced

1 leek, sliced (optional)

1 tsp tomato purée (optional)

2 cups stock or water

Preheat oven to 350°F.

Trim off excess fat from the lamb, season with salt, and lay in the sprigs of rosemary over the joint. Place in a roasting pan and put in the oven for 15 minutes to seal. Remove from the oven and transfer to a large casserole dish. Add the vegetables, tomato purée, and stock/water and cover with the lid. Return to the oven, reducing the temperature to 300°F and cook for another 2 hours, until very tender.

Place the lamb on a serving dish with the vegetables and keep warm. Strain off the juices, skimming off any excess fat, and serve in a jug. This can be thickened with sago, tapioca, or any permissible flour.

Shoulder of lamb with apricot, raisin, and oat stuffing

Good for: Elimination Diet, Day 16

Serves 4

FOR THE STUFFING

1½ cups fresh apricots, chopped

⅓ cup raisins

⅔ cup oat flakes

2 tsp fresh tarragon, parsley, or chosen herb

sea salt

1 tsp tapioca flour

1 cup stock or water

1 boned shoulder of lamb

Preheat the oven to 350°F and reduce to 325°F after the first 15 minutes.

For the stuffing, put the apricots, raisins, oats, and seasoning in a bowl and bind together with the tapioca and stock/water. Place the stuffing into the cavity of the meat and tie with string or secure with skewers. Roast for 1½ to 2 hours and serve with gravy.

Creamy lamb with rye spaghetti

Good for: Elimination Diet, Day 20

Serves 4

1 cup lamb stock

1 lb lean lamb, cut into strips

1 large red pepper, deseeded and cut into 2" strips

1½ cups zucchini, cut into 2" strips

1 clove garlic

½ tsp ground rosemary

pinch of nutmeg

sea salt

1½ tbsp sago/tapioca/corn starch (optional)

1¼ cup sheep's milk yogurt

2¾ cup rye spaghetti, barley, or buckwheat pasta, cooked

Pour the stock into a saucepan and bring to a boil. Add the lamb, vegetables, and seasoning and cook gently for 15 minutes. Thicken with the sago flour/tapioca/corn starch if necessary. Just before serving, stir in the yogurt and serve with rye pasta.

Deviled lamb's kidneys

Good for: Preliminary Diet

Serves 4

4 lamb's kidneys

2½ tbsp gram flour (chickpea flour)

sea salt (optional)

1 cup lamb stock

Wash the kidneys in cold water. Dry and remove the cores. Cut into thin slices and roll each slice in the gram flour, sprinkled with a little salt if desired. Heat the stock in a pan, add the kidneys, and cook gently for 4 to 5 minutes

Moussaka

Good for: Elimination Diet, Day 24

Serves 4

4 large eggplant, sliced

sea salt

2 large onions, chopped

1 clove garlic, crushed

2 tbsp sesame seed oil

1 lb lean minced lamb or 3 cups aduki beans, sprouted and cooked

1 cup tomatoes, skinned and chopped

1 green pepper, deseeded and chopped

1 tbsp tomato purée

½ tsp oregano

sea salt or kelp

FOR THE SAUCE

2 free-range eggs or soy egg replacer

1 cup goat's milk yogurt

½ tsp allspice or nutmeg

½ tsp ground mustard

½ tsp salt to taste

½ cup hard goat's cheese, grated

Preheat the oven to 325°F.

Sprinkle the eggplant slices with salt to remove bitterness. Leave for 30 minutes, drain, and dry on kitchen paper. Steam or boil in a little water until tender and set to one side.

Sauté the onions and garlic in oil and water until transparent. Add the lamb/aduki beans, tomatoes, pepper, and flavorings and cook for 10 minutes. Using a well-oiled shallow ovenproof baking dish, arrange the eggplant slices and the lamb/aduki bean mixture in layers.

For the sauce, beat together the eggs and yogurt and add the spices and seasoning. Pour over the top and sprinkle with grated cheese. Bake for 30 to 40 minutes.

Chili con carne

Good for: Elimination Diet, Day 24

Serves 4

2 cups stock

1 lb organic lean beef steak, cut into cubes

2 onions, chopped

2 cloves garlic, crushed

½ tsp cayenne pepper

1 tsp oregano

sea salt

6 tomatoes, skinned and chopped

2¾ cup red kidney beans, sprouted and cooked

1 tbsp barley or rice flour

Pour the stock into a heavy-based saucepan and bring to a boil. Add all the ingredients except the tomatoes and kidney beans. Cover and cook for 1 hour or until the meat is tender.

Add the tomatoes and kidney beans and cook for another 15 minutes. Mix the barley flour with a little cold water and stir into the juices to thicken.

Pork, apple, and chestnut pie

Good for: Elimination Diet, Day 13

Serves 4

FOR THE FILLING

8 ounces minced pork

1¾ cups chestnuts, cooked and broken into pieces

1¾ cups Cox's apples, peeled and sliced

4 quail's eggs or 2½ tbsp soy egg replacer, beaten

½ cup stock

1 tsp fresh thyme or ½ tsp dried

sea salt

FOR THE SWEET POTATO AND BUCKWHEAT PASTRY

⅔ cup sweet potato, baked and mashed

⅓ cup buckwheat flour

⅓ cup soy flour

½ cup olive oil

1 tsp baking powder (wheat free)

sea salt

water to mix

1 egg, beaten

Preheat the oven to 325°F and line and grease a 8" pie tin.

For the filling, mix together all the ingredients.

For the pastry, mix the ingredients and form into a firm dough. Roll out two-thirds of the pastry and line the base of the pie tin. Prick the base and spread with the filling. Cover with the remaining pastry and seal the edges. Brush with a little beaten egg and pierce the lid of the pie to allow steam to escape. Bake for 50 minutes and serve hot or cold.

Pork tenderloin with prune, anchovy, and almond stuffing

Good for: Elimination Diet, Day 21

Serves 4

18 large prunes

8 anchovy fillets

8 blanched almonds

2 outdoor reared/organic pork tenderloins

2½ cups vegetable or bone marrow stock

1 tbsp arrowroot

salt

Soak the prunes overnight and remove pits before using.

Preheat the oven to 350°F.

To stuff eight prunes, wrap an anchovy fillet around a blanched almond and fill the cavity of the prune.

To prepare the tenderloins, slit down one long side, just over halfway through, and open out. Lay the stuffed prunes on one opened out tenderloin. Lay the second tenderloin on top and tie together at intervals with string. Place in an ovenproof casserole and bake for 40 minutes, reducing the oven temperature to 325°F after the first 20 minutes.

Cook the remaining prunes for 1 to 2 minutes. Drain and place on one side, keeping the liquid to add to the sauce.

Remove the pork tenderloin from the casserole, carve into slices, and arrange on a hot serving dish. Use the cooking juices, stock, seasoning, and the prune juice to make a sauce, and thicken with arrowroot. Pour over the meat, and garnish with the remaining prunes.

Sweet and sour vegetables/pork

Good for: Elimination Diet, Day 21

Serves 4

FOR THE SWEET AND SOUR SAUCE

½ cup water

2 tsp corn starch/tapioca/sago

2½ tbsp soy sauce

2½ tbsp wine vinegar

1 tbsp clear honey

1 tbsp tomato purée

1 lb lean organic pork, cut into strips (optional)

1½ cups zucchini, sliced

1 cup water chestnuts

¾ cup baby corn

¾ cup sugar peas

1 carrot, cut into julienne strips

1 red/green pepper, deseeded and sliced

½ cucumber, diced

2½ tbsp sesame seed oil

To make the sweet and sour sauce, cream together the corn starch and water, mix in the remaining ingredients, and pour into a saucepan. Gently cook, stirring all the time, until the sauce thickens.

For the pork and vegetables, heat some water in the bottom of the wok and cook the pork. Add the vegetables in order of cooking time until just tender. Add the sweet and sour sauce, tossing the vegetables until all are coated and the sauce thickens. Just before serving, stir in the sesame seed oil.

Pork and pineapple kebabs

Good for: Rotation Diet, Day 2

Serves 4

1½ lbs lean organic pork, cut into 1" cubes

1 pineapple, skinned and cut into cubes

2 green peppers, deseeded and cut into ¾" pieces

8 bay leaves

2 tsp freshly chopped thyme

sea salt

Thread the pork, pineapple cubes, green pepper pieces, and bay leaves on to four long skewers. Sprinkle with thyme and salt; and place the kebabs on an oiled grill rack. Grill over medium heat for 10 to 15 minutes, turning frequently.

Pig's liver and onions

Good for: Rotation Diet, Day 2

Serves 4

2½ tbsp olive oil

3 onions, sliced

1 lb organic pig's liver, thinly sliced

1 tbsp fine oatmeal

sea salt

1 cup pork or vegetable stock or water

1 tsp corn starch

Warm the oil with a little water in a heavy-based frying pan. Cool fry the onions until transparent and place on a serving dish and keep warm.

Roll the slices of liver in the oatmeal seasoned with salt, and gently fry on both sides until just cooked (2 to 3 minutes). Place on top of the onions.

To make a gravy, add the stock to the pan, adding a little corn starch mixed with cold water if necessary.

Meatballs in tomato sauce

Good for: Rotation Diet, Day 2

Serves 4

FOR THE SAUCE

6 fresh tomatoes, skinned and chopped

1 pepper, deseeded and diced

2 spring onions, chopped

1 clove garlic, crushed

1 tsp basil

½ tsp cayenne pepper

sea salt

2 cups stock or water

FOR THE MEATBALLS

1 lb minced meat (pork or venison)

1 large onion, chopped (not fried)

2 cloves garlic, crushed

2½ tbsp tomato purée

2½ tbsp fine oatmeal or corn meal

1 tsp ginger grated

½ tsp ground cardamom

½ tsp chili powder (optional)

sea salt

For the sauce, cook the vegetables in the stock/water for 15 minutes until tender.

For the meatballs, mix together all the ingredients either by hand or in a food mixer, and mold into approximately eight meatballs. Bring the stock to a boil and add the meatballs. Pour over the tomato sauce and simmer gently for 30 minutes.

Roast pork/wild boar with juniper

Good for: Rotation Diet, Day 2

Serves 4

1 tbsp fine oatmeal

2½ tbsp freshly chopped sage

10 juniper berries, crushed

2 cloves garlic, crushed

sea salt

2 lbs boned loin of organically reared pork

Preheat the oven to 350°F.

Mix together the oatmeal, sage, juniper berries, garlic, and seasoning. Trim off the skin and excess fat from the pork, and cut some deep slashes in the top and sides. Place in a roasting tray, and press in the herb and juniper mixture. Roast for approximately 1 hour until thoroughly cooked.

Wild boar cutlets with mushroom sauce

Good for: Elimination Diet, Day 13

Serves 4

4 to 6 wild boar loan cutlets, trimmed

2½ cups stock

1½ cups small turnips, diced

1 tsp ground mustard seeds

sea salt

1 cup button mushrooms

sago or tapioca flour

Grill the cutlets on both sides to seal the juices. Place in a pan with the stock, turnips, and seasoning and bring to a boil. Cover and simmer for 30 minutes and then add the mushrooms. Cook for another 5 minutes. Thicken the juices with a little sago or tapioca flour.

Fruit-roasted leg of wild boar

Good for: Elimination Diet, Day 25

Serves 8 to 10

FOR THE FRUIT COATING

1 cup dried apricots, finely chopped

1 cup dried prunes, finely chopped

10 juniper berries, crushed

grated zest and juice of 1 orange

2½ tbsp oatmeal

1 tsp allspice

sea salt

3½–4 lbs whole leg of wild boar

2½ cups prune juice

arrowroot (optional)

Preheat the oven to 350°F and reduce to 325°F after the first 20 minutes.

Mix together the ingredients for the fruit coating, using a little of the prune juice to bind if necessary.

Trim off the skin and any excess fat from the leg and place, inner side down, in a well-oiled roasting pan. Coat the upper surface with the fruit mixture, pressing it down evenly as you go. Pour the prune juice around the joint and cook for 40 minutes per 1 lb weight, basting with the prune juice from time to time until thoroughly cooked.

Transfer to a warm serving dish. Add some water to the roasting pan and boil up the juices. Skim off any fat, thicken with arrowroot or similar flour if you wish, and serve with the meat.

FISH

Red mullet with seasoned rice stuffing

Good for: Preliminary Diet

Serves 4

4 red mullet, about 6 ounces each, cleaned and scaled

sea salt

FOR THE STUFFING

¾ cup long grain rice, cooked

⅓ cup pine nuts

⅓ cup golden raisins

¼ cup chopped olives (not in vinegar)

1 tsp ground lemongrass

1 tsp cilantro

sea salt

Preheat the oven to 350°F.

Mix together the ingredients for the stuffing and fill the cavity of each fish, and secure with a skewer.

Place the fish in a well-oiled baking pan, sprinkle with salt, and bake for 30 to 35 minutes.

Rolled flounder with spinach

Good for: Elimination Diet, Day 10

Serves 4

1.5 lbs spinach

4 fillets of flounder

½ cup corn or millet flour

½ cup ground cashew nuts

sea salt

sprigs of parsley, for garnishing

Preheat the oven to 325°F.

Thoroughly wash and steam the spinach in its own moisture until tender. Mash with a fork and place in a well-oiled casserole dish.

Cut the flounder filets in two, lengthways, and roll up each half, securing with a toothpick. Arrange on top of the spinach and sprinkle with a mixture of millet flour, ground cashew nuts, and sea salt. Cover and cook for 30 minutes. Serve garnished with parsley.

Fisherman's pie

Good for: Rotation Diet, Day 4

Serves 4

1 lb fillet of cod or similar fish

1 cup sheep's or goat's milk

sea salt

1 tbsp tapioca flour

2¼ cups yam, cooked and mashed

Preheat the oven to 325°F.

Place the fish in a pan and cover with the milk and a pinch of salt. Bring to a boil and simmer very gently for 4 to 5 minutes until just cooked. Strain off the milk and place the fish in a pie dish.

Mix the flour with a little water and add to the milk. Cook, stirring until the sauce thickens and pour over the fish. Top with mashed yam and bake for 30 minutes.

Buckwheat and walnut coated herrings

Good for: Rotation Diet, Day 4

Serves 4

4 herrings

FOR THE TOPPING

1 cup buckwheat flakes

⅓ cup walnuts, finely chopped

½ cup sheep's yogurt

1 tsp ground mustard seeds

1 tbsp butter (optional)

sea salt or kelp

Wash and scale the herrings and cut off the heads. Slit the herrings open and remove the guts and backbones. Grill the herrings on both sides until almost cooked.

For the topping, mix together the ingredients and spread over the cutlets. Grill for another minute.

Grilled halibut with anchovy butter

Good for: Rotation Diet, Day 4

Serves 4

4 halibut steaks

FOR THE ANCHOVY BUTTER

2.5 ounces anchovy fillets

½ cup unsalted butter

Preheat and grease the grill pan and grill the halibut for 6 to 8 minutes until just cooked through. There should be no need to turn.

To prepare the butter, rinse and dry the anchovies. Chop finely and rub through a sieve. Beat into the butter, form into butter pats, and serve with the halibut.

Fresh salmon with raspberry coulis

Good for: Elimination Diet, Day 14

Serves 4

4 wild salmon fillets

sea salt

1¾ cups fresh raspberries

½ cup water

1 tbsp fruit sugar

Sprinkle the salmon fillets with salt and poach for 4 to 5 minutes.

Place the raspberries in a saucepan with the water and fruit sugar and bring to a boil. Simmer until the raspberries begin to break up. Blend, strain, and serve with the salmon.

Salmon and tomato fish cakes

Good for: Elimination Diet, Day 26

Serves 4

8 ounces flaked, cooked salmon

1 cup cooked and mashed potato or yam

2 to 3 tomatoes, skinned and chopped

1½ tbsp capers, chopped

1 onion, finely chopped

1 tsp arrowroot or tapioca flour

1 tbsp lemon juice or 1 tsp lemongrass

1 tsp thyme

sea salt or kelp

2½ tbsp corn or millet flour for coating

Preheat the oven to 325°F.

Mix all the ingredients together and mold into four fish cakes and roll in the corn flour. Bake for 25 minutes.

Prawn or tofu chow mein

Good for: Elimination Diet, Day 26

Serves 4

10" wakame seaweed

8 ounces vermicelli (rice noodles)

1 cup bean sprouts

1 cup water chestnuts, sliced

1 cup organic mushrooms, sliced

2 carrots, thinly sliced diagonally

½ cup vegetable stock

12 ounces shelled prawns or 4½ cups tofu, cut into squares

1 tbsp tamari soy sauce

1 tbsp organic white wine (optional)

sesame seed oil, for garnishing

Wash and soak the wakame seaweed for 10 minutes. Drain and cut into 1" pieces. The soaking water may be used to cook the noodles. Bring the water to a boil and cook the vermicelli until just soft. Drain well and place on a serving dish and keep warm.

Heat some water in a wok or saucepan and cook the vegetables for 5 minutes. Add the stock and bring to a boil. Add the prawns, seaweed, soy sauce, and wine and cook for another 3 minutes. Place on the serving dish in the center of the noodles and sprinkle with sesame seed oil.

Grilled trout fillets with tropical fruit

Good for: Rotation Diet, Day 1

Serves 4

1 large mango

4 pieces of trout fillet (not farmed)

sea salt

1 tsp ground coriander

1 star fruit

2½ tbsp fresh cilantro, chopped, for garnishing

To prepare the mango, hold upright and take a slice off each side, cutting down as near to the stone as possible, then cutting the smaller pieces off the ends. Skin and cut into matchstick pieces.

Place the trout in a grill pan, sprinkle with salt and ground coriander, and grill for 5 to 7 minutes. Arrange on a bed of the mango and sliced star fruit, and garnish with chopped cilantro.

Stuffed squid

Good for: Rotation Diet, Day 1

Serves 4

2 lbs small squid, cleaned and prepared

FOR THE STUFFING

1 cup breadcrumbs or cooked millet

2 ribs celery, finely diced

2½ tbsp fresh parsley, chopped

3½ tbsp sesame seed oil

rind of 1 lemon

sea salt or kelp

3 carrots, cut into matchsticks

1 cup vegetable stock

chopped parsley for garnishing

lemon wedges for garnishing

Preheat the oven to 325°F.

Mix together the ingredients for the stuffing, and stuff the squid bodies with the mixture. Sew up or fasten the opening with a toothpick. Place in an ovenproof dish with the carrots, and pour over the stock. Bake for 45 minutes and serve hot with a sprinkling of parsley and lemon wedges.

Seafood paella

Good for: Elimination Diet, Day 22

Serves 6 to 8

1 lb fresh mussels

1 bay leaf

4¼ cups water or vegetable stock

2½ tbsp olive oil

1 onion, peeled and chopped

2 cloves garlic

1½ cups long-grain rice

sea salt

1 tsp ground lemongrass

Saffron

1 cup tomatoes, skinned and chopped

1 red pepper, deseeded and sliced

¾ cup peas

1 lb small squid, cleaned, prepared and cut into rings

6 ounces prepared scallops

FOR THE GARNISHING

1¼ cups black olives (preservative free)

1 lemon cut into wedges

2 tsp fresh cilantro, chopped

Scrub the mussels, removing the threadlike beards and discarding any that do not close when tapped. Place in a pan with water and a bay leaf and cook for 5 minutes until the shells open. Strain off the liquid and make up to 4¼ cups with water or vegetable stock. Reserve 8 to 10 mussels in their shells, and shell the rest, discarding any that have not opened.

Warm the oil and a little water in a large shallow saucepan or paella pan, and sauté the onion and garlic until soft. Stir in the rice and cook for 1 to 2 minutes. Add the stock, salt, lemongrass, and saffron, bring to a boil and cook for 15 minutes. Stir in the tomatoes, red pepper, peas, squid, scallops, and shelled mussels, and cook for 4 to 5 minutes until the rice is tender. Serve garnished with mussels in their shells, black olives, wedges of lemon, and a sprinkling of cilantro.

VEGETARIAN

Spanish omelette

Good for: Elimination Diet, Day 27

Serves 4

2½ tbsp olive oil
1 onion, chopped
2 cloves garlic, crushed
2 zucchini, thinly sliced
2 tomatoes skinned, deseeded, and chopped
1 tsp oregano
sea salt
4 free-range chicken eggs

Warm the olive oil and a little water in a pan and sauté the onions
until soft. Add the garlic, zucchini, tomatoes, and seasoning, cover
the pan, and cook gently for 7 to 10 minutes.

Beat the eggs and stir into the vegetables. Cook over gentle heat
for 2 to 3 minutes until the underside is cooked. Place the pan
under a preheated grill and cook the top of the omelette for another
2 to 3 minutes until set. Cut into quarters and serve.

Millet and cashew nut risotto

Good for: Elimination Diet, Day 10

Serves 4

2 ribs celery, sliced
8 ounces millet, cooked
¾ cup cashew nuts
½ cup black olives (preservative free)

Blanche the sliced celery by immersing in boiling water for
30 seconds. Mix the ingredients together and serve hot or cold.

Millet, lentil, and brazil nut loaf

Good for: Preliminary Diet; Elimination Diet, Day 26

Serves 4

1¼ cups millet

1¼ cups green lentils, sprouted

1 cup vegetable stock or mineral water

1 tbsp tapioca flour

1¼ cups Brazil nuts, roughly chopped

2 ribs celery, diced

1 tbsp sage

sea salt

Preheat the oven to 325°F.

Cook the millet and lentils in the stock/water for 15 minutes and mix with the rest of the ingredients in a food mixer or with a wooden spoon. Oil a loaf tin or deep pie dish and press the mixture in well. Bake for 45 minutes or until the top of the loaf is brown and firm to the touch. Serve hot or cold.

Barley, cashew, and vegetable loaf

Good for: Preliminary Diet; Elimination Diet, Day 25; Rotation Diet, Day 1

Serves 4

2¼ cups pot barley, cooked

1¼ cups shiitake mushrooms, diced

1¼ cups cashew nuts, chopped

2 carrots, grated

2½ tbsp barley flour

2½ tbsp freshly chopped cilantro

½ cup stock or water

sea salt or 1 tsp barley miso

Preheat the oven to 325°F.

Mix together all the ingredients and turn into a lined loaf tin. Bake for about 50 minutes until firm.

Sweet potato and seafood bakes

Good for: Preliminary Diet; Elimination Diet, Day 6

Serves 4

1½ cups sweet potato

8 ounces tuna fish, cooked

basil

sea salt

quinoa flour

Preheat the oven to 325°F.

Cook the sweet potatoes by boiling or baking. Do not fry. A large sweet potato weighing 1 lb will take 1 hour to cook at 325°F.

Mix together the sweet potato and tuna fish. Add the basil and salt. Make into cakes and roll each one in the quinoa flour. Bake for 20 minutes, turning once.

For larger quantities, the mixture may be formed into a roll on a lightly floured board and cut into slices before shaping and flouring. Useful for freezing.

Zucchini bakes may be made in a similar way, substituting grated zucchini for tuna fish.

Aduki bean burgers

Good for: Rotation Diet, Day 3

Serves 4

3⅓ cups sprouted and cooked aduki beans

1 cup cooked organic short grain rice

¾ cup ground almonds

1 tbsp sago flour

1 tsp freshly chopped tarragon

sea salt

Mash together all the ingredients and shape into burgers or use a burger press. Grill for 4 to 5 minutes on each side under low to moderate heat.

Brazil nut bean burgers

Good for: Elimination Diet, Day 9

Serves 4

3 cups black-eyed beans, sprouted and cooked

1⅔ cups Brazil nuts, soaked and chopped

2½ cups buckwheat flakes

2½ tbsp safflower oil

1 tsp dried sage

sea salt

1 tsp millet flour

Preheat the oven to 325°F.

Mix together all the ingredients, adding a little water if necessary, and mold into burgers or use a burger press. Roll in millet flour and bake for 20 minutes.

Brazil nut roast

Good for: Rotation Diet, Day 2

Serves 4

1⅓ cups corn flour

1 cup oatflakes

2 cups Brazil nuts, chopped

1 cup zucchini, grated

2 onions, finely chopped

1 cup water

1 tbsp freshly chopped sage

sea salt

1 tbsp olive oil

Preheat the oven to 325°F.

Line a 2 lb loaf tin with wax paper. Mix together all the ingredients, adding more water if necessary, and turn into the tin. Bake for 1 hour until firm to the touch.

This recipe may also be used for burgers and stuffing.

Quinoa nut roast

Good for: Preliminary Diet

Serves 6 to 8

3⅓ cups quinoa, cooked

2½ cups carrots, grated

¾ cup zucchini, grated

2 ribs celery, chopped

¾ cup ground almonds

⅓ cup whole almonds, chopped

¾ cup sunflower seeds

¼ cup olive oil

½ cup vegetable stock or mineral water

2½ tbsp sago flour

fresh sage or tarragon, chopped or 1 tsp dried

sea salt

Preheat the oven to 325°F.

Line one or two loaf tins with wax paper. Mix all the ingredients together and turn into the tins. Bake for 1 hour. A soup may be used as a sauce.

Apricot and almond pilaf

Good for: Preliminary Diet; Rotation Diet, Day 3;
Elimination Diet, Day 8

Serves 4

2 cups sorghum/quinoa (use quinoa on Rotation Diet, Day 3)
8½ cups mineral water (sorghum) or 4¼ cups mineral water (quinoa)
sea salt
1 cup fresh apricots, cut into quarters
1 cup almonds
¼ cup sunflower seeds, for garnishing
2½ tbsp sunflower oil

Rinse the sorghum and place in a saucepan with the water and a
pinch of salt. Bring to a boil and simmer for 1 hour (30 minutes for
quinoa) until soft adding the apricots during the last 5 minutes of
cooking time. Cut the almonds in half, lengthways, and add the
sorghum, together with the tarragon. Serve, garnished with the
sunflower seeds, and pour over the sunflower oil.

Tempeh or tofu stir-fry

Good for: Rotation Diet, Day 3
Serves 4

2 cups snow peas, topped and tailed
2 cups green beans, sliced
1¾ cups mung bean sprouts
2 heads Belgian endive, sliced
2¾ cup tempeh or tofu, cut into cubes
1 tbsp Tamari soy sauce
2½ tbsp sunflower oil
⅔ cup almonds, cut lengthways, for garnishing

Heat a little water in a wok and cook the vegetables in order of
cooking time. Add the tempeh or tofu and soy sauce. Stir in the
oil and garnish with almonds.

Vegetable goulash with dumplings

Good for: Elimination Diet, Day 12

Serves 4

1 cup tomatoes, skinned and chopped

1 cup green beans, cut into 1" lengths

¾ cup potatoes, cut into even-sized chunks

2 carrots, sliced

2 ribs celery

2 cups water

1 tbsp tomato purée

sprig of rosemary or thyme

sea salt or kelp

2½ tbsp sunflower oil

FOR THE BARLEY DUMPLINGS
(see page 193)

Place all the vegetables and the water, in a heavy-based saucepan and bring to a boil. Add the tomato purée, seasoning, and dumplings, and cook gently for 40 minutes. Remove the sprigs, stir in the oil, and serve.

Smoked tofu and mushroom kebabs

Good for: Elimination Diet, Day 13

Serves 4

2 cups button mushrooms

4 wooden skewers

2¾ cups smoked tofu

fresh herbs, for garnishing

French dressing (see page 197)

Cut the mushrooms into halves and use them raw or quickly blanched in boiling water. Cut the tofu into 1" cubes and thread onto a skewer alternating each cube with a mushroom. Arrange on a serving dish on a bed of lettuce leaves and pour over the salad dressing.

Green pepper and pine nut pizza

Good for: Elimination Diet, Day 12

Serves 4

FOR THE DOUGH

2 cups barley flour (or rice flour)
1¼ cups rutabaga, cooked and mashed
½ cup olive oil
sea salt

FOR THE SAUCE

1 onion, peeled and chopped
1 garlic clove, peeled and chopped
2 cups fresh tomatoes, skinned and chopped
1 zucchini, grated
1 large green pepper, deseeded and sliced
2 tbsp tomato purée
sea salt

FOR THE TOPPING

⅓ cup pine nuts
6 black olives stoned and halved
1 tsp oregano

Preheat the oven to 325°F.

To prepare the dough, mix together all the ingredients and mold into four individual rounds, or press into a well-oiled rectangular baking tray.

For the sauce, cook the onion and garlic for 3 to 4 minutes until soft. Add the tomatoes, zucchini, green pepper, tomato purée, and salt, and spoon onto the dough bases.

Top with pine nuts and olives, and sprinkle with oregano. Bake for 20 to 25 minutes.

Breadfruit with ginger and green peppers

Good for: Elimination Diet, Day 14

Serves 4

1 breadfruit

2 green peppers, sliced

1 large pear, peeled, cored and sliced

3 cardamom pods, crushed

1 tsp ginger, grated

2 cups water

1 tbsp tahini

Peel and core the breadfruit and cut into chunks. Steam for 30 minutes until tender.

For the sauce, put the peppers and pear in a pan with the cardamom pods, ginger, and water, and cook until soft. Add the tahini and blend until smooth. Place the breadfruit on a serving dish and pour over the sauce.

Cashew nut and celery flan

Good for: Rotation Diet, Day 1

Serves 4

FOR THE PASTRY

¼ cup sesame seed oil

1½ cups wheat or barley flour

water to mix

pinch of salt

FOR THE SAUCE

2½ cups cashew nut milk, or vegetable stock

⅓ cup wheat or barley flour

sea salt

FOR THE FILLING

4 ribs celery, diced and cooked

1 cup cashew nuts

2½ tbsp parsley, freshly chopped

Preheat the oven to 325°F.

For the pastry, rub the oil into the flour and form into a firm dough with a little water and a pinch of salt. Roll out the pastry and line a 8 inch flan dish. Bake blind (cover with wax paper and weighed with baking beans) for 25 minutes until the pastry is evenly cooked.

For the sauce, heat the cashew nut milk/stock in a saucepan. Mix the flour with a little cold water and stir into the milk, and stir briskly until the sauce thickens. Season to taste.

For the filling, spread the celery and cashew nuts evenly over the pastry and sprinkle with parsley. Pour over the sauce and bake for another 25 minutes.

Green pepper and eggplant flan

Good for: Elimination Diet, Day 16; Rotation Diet, Day 2

Serves 4

FOR THE PASTRY CASE

1¼ cups fine oatmeal

¾ cup cooked mashed potato

½ cup olive oil

pinch of salt

FOR THE FILLING

2 eggplant, thinly sliced

sea salt

2 green peppers, thinly sliced

8–10 pitted olives (optional)

FOR THE SAUCE

1 cup vegetable stock or water

1 onion, finely chopped

1 tbsp corn starch

1 tbsp freshly chopped basil

sea salt

Preheat the oven to 325°F.

To prepare the flan case, mix together the ingredients using a little cold water to make a firm dough. Roll out between two sheets of wax paper or tough polythene and mold into a 9 inch flan dish.

For the filling, sprinkle the sliced eggplant with salt and leave for 30 minutes. Drain and dry on kitchen paper (this removes the bitterness). Steam or boil in a little water for 3 to 5 minutes until just tender, and arrange in the flan case with the green peppers and olives.

For the sauce, bring the stock/water to a boil and cook the onion until soft. Mix the corn starch with a little cold water and stir into the stock to thicken the sauce. Add the basil and salt, and pour into the flan case. Bake for 40 minutes.

Spinach and lentil flan

Good for: Rotation Diet, Day 3

Serves 4

FOR THE RICE PASTRY

1¼ cups rice flour

½ cup soy or gram flour

½ cup sunflower seed oil

½ cup water

FOR THE FILLING

1½ cups vegetable stock or water

2⅓ cups brown lentils, sprouted

sea salt

3⅔ cup spinach

½ tsp ground fenugreek

sunflower seeds for garnishing

Preheat the oven to 325°F.

Mix together all the pastry ingredients. Unlike pastry made with wheat, this dough does not roll easily, so it is better to pat down evenly into a 9 inch flan dish that has been well oiled.

For the filling, bring the stock/water to a boil and add the lentils and salt. Cook for 20 to 25 minutes until the lentils form a purée. Wash the spinach, then drain and cook it in its own juices in a covered pan. Drain, chop, and mix with the lentils and ground fenugreek. Spread the mixture in the flan case and bake for 25 minutes. Garnish with a sprinkling of sunflower seeds.

Feta cheese and cabbage pie

Good for: Rotation Diet, Day 4

Serves 4

FOR THE PASTRY CASE

2¼ cups sweet potato baked, skinned and mashed

½ cup butter

1 cup tapioca flour

FOR THE FILLING

1¼ cups Feta or goat's cheese

2¼ cups cabbage, finely shredded

Preheat the oven to 300°F.

For the pastry, mix together the sweet potato, butter, and tapioca flour and form into a dough. Take two-thirds and press into a 9 inch ovenproof flan dish. Fill with layers of thinly sliced Feta cheese and finely shredded cabbage.

On a floured board using tapioca flour to stop sticking, roll out the remaining dough to fit the top. Bake for 45 minutes until the top is crisp.

Vegetable and lentil dal

Good for: Elimination Diet, Day 22

Serves 4

2 cups stock or water

1⅔ cups green lentils, sprouted

1 onion, chopped

1 pepper, deseeded and chopped

2 ribs celery

2 carrots, chopped

1 tsp ground cumin

1 tsp ground coriander

2 bay leaves

sea salt or kelp

Pour the stock/water into a saucepan and bring to a boil. Add the lentils, vegetables, and seasoning and return to a boil. Simmer for 20 minutes until all the vegetables are tender. Remove the bay leaves and serve on a bed of millet or bulgur wheat.

Cauliflower and chickpea curry

Good for: Elimination Diet, Day 15

Serves 4

2½ tbsp olive oil

1 large onion, sliced

1 tsp ginger, grated

2 cloves garlic, crushed

2 tsp curry powder (wheat free)

½ cup creamed coconut

1 tbsp tomato purée

1¼ cups potatoes, diced

4½ cups vegetable stock or water

2¼ cups chickpeas, sprouted and cooked

1 small cauliflower, broken into florets

1 green pepper, deseeded and sliced

2 ribs celery, chopped

1 tbsp lemon juice

sea salt

Warm the oil and a little water in a pan, and gently cook the onions until transparent but not brown. Add the ginger, garlic, and curry powder and sauté for 1 to 2 minutes; then add the coconut, tomato purée stock, and potatoes. Bring to a boil and simmer for 5 minutes. Add the remaining ingredients and cook for another 15 minutes until the vegetables are tender.

Sweet potato and parsnip bakes

Good for: Elimination Diet, Day 23

Serves 4

2¼ cups cooked sweet potato, mashed

1 cup cooked parsnips, mashed

1 large onion, finely chopped

1 clove garlic, crushed

1 tsp ground mustard seed

1 tbsp fresh parsley, chopped

sea salt

1 tbsp sesame seeds for coating

Preheat the oven to 325°F.

Mix together the ingredients and form into potato cakes. Roll in the sesame seeds and bake for 25 minutes.

Buckwheat pasta with broccoli and walnuts

Good for: Rotation Diet, Day 4

Serves 4

8 ounces buckwheat spaghetti or pasta spirals (wheat free)

4 cups broccoli

sea salt

1⅔ cups walnuts, presoaked and chopped

2½ tbsp walnut oil

½ cup freshly grated Parmesan cheese or walnuts (optional)

Cook the pasta in plenty of boiling, salted water until al dente (tender without being too soft). Drain and keep warm on a serving dish.

Cut the florets from the broccoli, and cut the stalks diagonally across to make oval shapes (the stalks may be discarded and used in soup if you wish). Add a sprinkling of salt, and steam for 4 to 5 minutes until the florets turn a rich green, taking care not to overcook. Add the cooked broccoli and the walnuts to the pasta and spoon over the oil. May be served with walnuts or grated Parmesan cheese.

Root vegetable crumble

Good for: Elimination Diet, Day 25

Serves 4

FOR THE FILLING

1 cup vegetable stock

2½ cups of the following vegetables, diced: yam/sweet potato, turnip, carrots,
  parsnip, rutabaga

2 leeks, sliced (optional)

2 ribs celery, sliced

6 inch strip kombu seaweed

1 bay leaf

pinch of nutmeg

2 tsp arrowroot or corn starch

sea salt

FOR THE CRUMBLE

½ cup olive oil

1¼ cups barley, rye, or wheat flour

⅓ cup chestnut flour

½ cup sunflower seeds, chopped

½ cup rolled oats

½ cup hazelnuts, chopped

1 tbsp chopped parsley

sea salt

Preheat the oven to 325°F.

For the filling, pour the stock into a saucepan. Bring to a boil and
add the vegetables and seasoning. Return to a boil and then cover and
simmer until tender. Mix the arrowroot with a little cold water and
add to the vegetables to thicken the juices. Remove the bay leaf and
place the vegetable mixture in an ovenproof dish.

Make the crumble by lightly working the oil into the flour with your
fingertips. Add the seeds, nuts, oats, and parsley, then season and mix
together. Sprinkle over the vegetables and bake for 25 to 30 minutes.

Kedgeree

Good for: Elimination Diet, Day 26

Serves 4

1 large onion, peeled and chopped

2 cloves garlic, crushed

1 tsp ginger, mashed, or ½ tsp ground ginger

1 green pepper, deseeded and chopped

1 lb cooked flaked cod, haddock, or other saltwater fish

¾ cup whole-meal rice, cooked

2 tsp turmeric

juice of 1 lemon

sea salt or kelp

2 tbsp sesame seed oil

1 tbsp freshly chopped parsley for garnishing

Gently cook the onion, garlic, ginger, and pepper in a little water until soft. Stir in the fish, rice, and seasonings and when thoroughly mixed and cooked through, turn onto a serving dish. Stir in the oil and garnish with parsley.

Millet croquettes

Good for: Rotation Diet, Day 1

Serves 4

8 ounces millet, cooked

3 ribs celery, diced

3 carrots, grated

2 tbsp millet flour

1 to 2 tbsp tahini

1 tbsp fresh parsley, chopped

½ cup water

sea salt or kelp

½ cup sesame seeds, for coating

Preheat the oven to 300°F.

Mix together all the ingredients and form into croquettes. Roll in the sesame seeds and bake for 25 minutes.

Baked beans in tomato sauce

Good for: Elimination Diet, Day 20

Serves 4

3 cups haricot beans, soaked and sprouted

1 carrot, diced

1 rib celery, diced

1 onion, chopped

1 clove garlic, crushed

1 cup tomatoes skinned, deseeded, and chopped

1 tbsp tomato purée

2½ cups game stock or water

1 tsp ground cumin

1 tbsp chopped parsley

sea salt

Preheat the oven to 325°F. Place all the ingredients in a casserole dish and bake in the oven for 1½ hours.

Stuffed baked potatoes

Good for: Elimination Diet, Days 15 & 28

Serves as many as you like

baked potatoes

FOR THE FILLINGS

fromage frais, celery, and chives

Cheddar cheese, mushrooms (chopped and cooked) and thyme

tuna fish with sweetcorn relish

salmon and tomato relish

Cheddar cheese and chutney

Preheat the oven to 375°F.

Scrub the potatoes and prick all over with a fork. Bake for about 1 hour until tender. Remove from the oven, cut a cross in the top, press open, and scoop out some of the soft center, placing it in a bowl. Mash with a filling and pile the mixture back into the potato and return to the oven for another 10 minutes to heat through.

Mixed vegetable terrine

Good for: Rotation Diet, Day 1

Serves 4

2 cups carrots

2 cups parsnips

2 cups celery root

3 tsp barley or wheat flour

3 tbsp sesame seed oil

sea salt

2 tbsp freshly chopped parsley

2 sheets nori seaweed

Preheat the oven to 325°F and line the base of a 3 lb loaf tin.

Cook the vegetables in separate saucepans and allow to cool. Blend each one separately in a blender, adding 1 tsp of flour, 1 tbsp of oil, and a pinch of salt to each. Blend the parsley with the celery root.

Carefully spoon the purées into the loaf tin starting with a parsnip layer, then the carrot, and finally the celery root, placing a sheet of nori seaweed between each layer. Bake for 1½ hours until firm. Cool and then refrigerate. Turn out of the tin when cold.

Polenta with tomato and pepper sauce

Good for: Rotation Diet, Day 2

Serves 4

6 fresh tomatoes, skinned and chopped

1 pepper, deseeded and diced

2 spring onions, chopped

1 clove garlic, crushed

1 tsp basil

½ tsp cayenne pepper

sea salt

FOR THE POLENTA

(see page 86)

Cook the vegetables and seasonings in a little water for 15 minutes until tender. Rub through a sieve or leave chunky. Cut the polenta into 2" squares. Serve hot with the tomato sauce.

Artichoke and three-bean casserole

Good for: Rotation Diet, Day 3

Serves 4

2½ cups vegetable stock or water

2 cups fresh green beans, cut into thirds

6 to 8 Jerusalem or globe artichoke hearts

2½ cups kidney beans, sprouted and cooked

2½ cups black-eyed beans, sprouted and cooked

½ tsp nutmeg

1 tbsp fresh tarragon or 2 tsp umeboshi purée

sea salt

Bring the stock/water to a boil and cook the French beans and artichoke hearts until tender. Add the remaining ingredients and flavorings and simmer for another 10 to 15 minutes.

Jerusalem artichokes may be used instead of globe artichokes.

Spinach roulade with chickpea and salsify filling

Good for: Rotation Diet, Day 3

Serves 4

3 cups spinach

4 eggs separated

⅓ cup rice flour

sea salt

FOR THE FILLING

3 cups salsify

3⅔ cups chickpeas, sprouted and cooked

sea salt

Preheat the oven to 350°F and line a baking pan with wax paper and brush with oil.

Wash the spinach and discard the stalks. Cook in its own juice for 4 to 5 minutes until tender. Cool and drain well; and place in a food mixer with the egg yolks, rice flour, and salt, and blend to form a smooth mixture. Whisk the egg whites in a clean bowl until they form stiff peaks. Fold into the spinach mixture and spread into the prepared tin. Cook for 20 minutes until firm.

For the filling, scrub the salsify and boil for 20 to 25 minutes. Peel and dice. Place in a food mixer with the cooked chickpeas and seasoning and blend until smooth adding some of the chickpea water to form a spreadable mixture. Turn the cooked roulade out onto a large sheet of wax paper, and peel off the lining paper. Spread with the chickpea filling and immediately roll up with the help of the paper. May be served hot or cold.

Rice

Good for: Preliminary Diet; Elimination Diet, Days 1-8

Serves 4

1 cup organic whole-grain rice

pinch of sea salt

2 cups mineral water

Rinse the rice and place in a saucepan with the salt. Pour over the water and bring to a boil. Turn the heat down, place the lid on the saucepan, and simmer gently for 30 minutes until all the water has been absorbed. Do not rinse, as this will wash away the nutrients. If there is too much water, strain and use the liquid in soup.

To cook presoaked rice, discard the water that was used for soaking, and follow the above procedure. The cooking time will be reduced to approximately 15 minutes.

Millet, quinoa, or amaranth

Good for: Preliminary Diet; Elimination Diet, Days 1–8

Serves 4

Follow the method for rice, reducing the amount of water to 1¾ cups.

Sorghum

Good for: Preliminary Diet

Serves 4

1 cup sorghum

4 cups mineral water

Cook as for rice, increasing the time to 1 hour.

Cardamom nut rice

Good for: Elimination Diet, Day 14

Serves 4

1 cup organic long grain rice

1 onion, chopped

1 clove garlic, crushed

1 tsp fresh ginger, finely grated

3 black cardamom pods, crushed

½ tsp ground cumin

½ tsp ground lemongrass

½ tsp turmeric

sea salt

2 cups vegetable stock or water

2 tbsp olive oil

½ cup pumpkin seeds

⅓ cup cashew nuts

⅓ cup almonds, blanched and halved lengthways

⅓ cup golden raisins

Put the rice in a pan with the onion, garlic, spices, salt and stock/water and bring to a boil. Cover and simmer for 25 to 30 minutes until the rice is cooked. Remove the cardamom pods from the rice and stir in the olive oil. Add the seeds, nuts, and sultanas and serve.

Lentils

Good for: Preliminary Diet

Serves 4

4 cups sprouted lentils

water

sea salt

Place the lentils in a saucepan with sufficient boiling water to cover, and a pinch of salt. Cook gently until tender. The cooking time will vary depending on how long the lentils have been sprouted.

Parsnip and walnut croquettes

Good for: Preliminary Diet; Elimination Diet, Day 7

Serves 4

1¼ cup cooked parsnips

1¼ cup cooked sweet potato or eddoe

2 ribs celery, finely diced

¾ cups walnuts, chopped

1 tsp tapioca flour

1 tbsp freshly chopped cilantro

sea salt

1 tbsp millet flour for coating

Preheat the oven to 325°F.

Mix together the ingredients and form into eight croquettes. Roll in millet flour and place on a baking tray and bake for 35 minutes.

Butternut squash with pine nuts

Good for: Elimination Diet, Day 10

Serves 4

3½ cups butternut squash, winter squash, or marrow

sea salt

1 tsp ground cumin or seeds

1 tsp lemongrass

1½ cups pine nuts

sprigs of fresh mint for garnishing

Peel the squash, cut in half lengthways, discard the seeds, and cut into crosswise slices. Steam or cook with a little boiling water, sprinkling in the salt, cumin, and lemongrass. Cook for 4 to 5 minutes until just tender. Arrange in a large shallow dish in overlapping layers. Sprinkle over the pine nuts and garnish with mint. Serve hot or cold.

Brussels sprouts with chestnuts

Good for: Elimination Diet, Day 11

Serves 4

3 cups whole cooked chestnuts or 1½ cups dried chestnuts, soaked and cooked
grated zest of 1 lemon
1 lb (about 4 cups) Brussels sprouts
1 leek, sliced
1 tbsp olive oil
sea salt
1 tbsp chopped parsley for garnishing

If you are using dried chestnuts, these will need to be soaked overnight before cooking. Cook the chestnuts and lemon zest in boiling salted water for 15 minutes until tender. Steam or boil the sprouts and leeks together with seasoning, for 5 to 7 minutes and drain. Add to the chestnuts and serve garnished with chopped parsley.

Stuffed papayas

Good for: Elimination Diet, Day 14

Serves 4

2 papayas
5 ounces trout (not farmed) or tofu
3 tbsp pine nuts
¼ cup wild rice, cooked
juice of 1 lime
iceberg lettuce for garnishing
alfalfa sprouts for garnishing

Cut the papayas in half and discard the seeds. Flake the trout and mix with the pine nuts and wild rice. Spoon the mixture into the hollow centers and pour over the lime juice. Place on individual plates and garnish with iceberg lettuce and alfalfa sprouts.

Roasted Jerusalem artichokes

Good for: Rotation Diet, Day 3

Serves 4

2⅔ cups Jerusalem artichokes, washed and scrubbed

dripping

Preheat the oven to 350°F.

Place the artichokes in a roasting pan. Pour over a little dripping from cooking game or poultry. Roast for about 45 minutes until golden.

Broccoli with ginger and macadamia nuts

Good for: Elimination Diet, Day 27

Serves 4

2½ cups broccoli

1 tsp ginger, grated

¼ cup macadamia nuts, cut into slivers

Cut the broccoli into small pieces, separating the florets and cutting the stems into diagonal slices. Steam with the ginger for 3 to 4 minutes until soft but still bright green. Sprinkle with the nuts and serve with couscous or millet.

Greek-style onions

Good for: Rotation Diet, Day 2

Serves 4

1 lb small pearl onions

1 cup stock or water

1 tbsp olive oil

2 tsp tomato purée

sprig of fresh thyme

sea salt

Blanch the onions in boiling water for 1 minute only, then drain and rinse in cold water. Remove the skins with a small knife or your fingers. Place the onions in a heavy-based saucepan with the stock/water, oil, tomato purée, thyme, and salt. Bring to a boil and simmer gently for 30 minutes. Remove the sprig of thyme and serve hot.

Baked vegetables

Good for: Rotation Diet, Day 2

Serves 4

1 red pepper, deseeded and halved

1 green pepper, deseeded and halved

1 large onion, skinned and quartered

6 whole cloves of garlic, skinned

3 to 4 zucchini, sliced lengthways

6 to 8 cherry tomatoes

1 bunch of asparagus, trimmed

2 tbsp olive oil or dripping

sea salt

herbs for garnishing, e.g., mint, basil, chives, oregano

Preheat the oven to 325°F.

Place the vegetables in a greased roasting pan with the oil or dripping and bake for 30 minutes. Sprinkle with salt and choice of herbs and serve hot.

Steamed vegetables

Good for: Preliminary Diet; Elimination Diet, Day 5

Serves 4

1½ cups broccoli florets

1½ cups swede, cut into julienne strips

1½ cups kohlrabi, diced

¾ cups turnip, diced

½ cup radishes, sliced

¾ cup cabbage, shredded

sea salt

Using a steamer or just a small amount of water, cook vegetables in order of cooking time and season to taste. May be served with a sprinkling of flaxseed oil.

Baked red cabbage

Good for: Elimination Diet, Day 25; Rotation Diet, Day 4

Serves 4

2 apples or pears

4½ cups red cabbage, shredded

4 to 5 cloves

½ tsp allspice

½ tsp mustard seeds

2½ tbsp cider vinegar (optional)

Preheat the oven to 325°F.

Peel the apples and cut into small segments. Immerse quickly in salt water to prevent browning. Place in a casserole dish with the cabbage, spices, and vinegar (if using), and bake for 1 hour. Remove the cloves and serve hot or cold.

Stuffed green peppers

Good for: Elimination Diet, Day 18

Serves 4

4 large green peppers

6 ounces minced lean lamb or sprouted and cooked aduki beans

¾ cups cooked rice

½ cup chopped almonds

¼ chopped olives

1 onion, chopped

1 tomato, peeled and diced

1 tsp ground coriander seeds

½ tsp ground cinnamon

sea salt

2 cups stock

Preheat the oven to 350°F.

Prepare the peppers for stuffing by removing a piece from the top of each and scooping out the seeds. Mix together all the ingredients, except the stock, and stuff each of the peppers. Place in a baking dish, replace the tops of the peppers, and pour over the stock. Bake for 1 hour, basting from time to time.

Bulgur wheat (cracked wheat)

Good for: Elimination Diet, Day 22

Serves 4

1 cup bulgur wheat

pinch of salt

2 cups boiling water

Place the bulgur wheat in a bowl with the salt and pour over a boiling water. Leave for 15 to 20 minutes until all the water has been absorbed.

Bubble and squeak nests

Good for: Elimination Diet, Day 27; Rotation Diet, Day 4

Serves 4

2¼ cups sweet potato or yam, grated

2¼ cups cabbage, shredded

¼ cup butter

⅓ cup amaranth or buckwheat flour

½ cup grated cheese (optional)

Preheat the oven to 300°F.

Mix together the grated vegetables and bind with the butter and flour. Divide into four mounds on a well-greased baking sheet and shape into nests. Top with grated cheese, (if using), and bake for 35 minutes.

Braised celery

Good for: Rotation Diet, Day 1

Serves 4

4 celery hearts, trimmed

2½ tbsp sesame seed oil

2½ tbsp flour

1¼ cups stock or water

sea salt

Preheat the oven to 325°F.

Place the celery in a well-oiled casserole dish. Warm the oil in a pan, stir in the flour, and cook for a few minutes. Gradually stir in the stock/water and cook until the sauce thickens, seasoning to taste. Pour over the celery and bake in the oven for 1 hour.

Barley dumplings

Good for: Elimination Diet, Day 12

Serves 4

1½ cups barley flour

1 tsp cream of tartar

½ tsp baking soda

⅓ cup dripping or olive oil

Mix together the ingredients with a little cold water and mould into four dumplings.

Baked plantains

Good for: Rotation Diet, Day 2

Serves 4

4 medium plantains

Preheat the oven to 325°F.

Bake the plantains in their skins for 30 minutes.

Millet, hazelnut and tofu croquettes

Good for: Elimination Diet, Day 19

Serves 4

1 cup millet flakes, cooked

1 cup silken tofu

¾ cups ground hazelnuts

1 tbsp tamari soy sauce

1 tbsp chopped fresh parsley

sea salt

2½ tbsp millet flour, for coating

Preheat the oven to 325°F.

Blend together all the ingredients and divide into eight croquettes. Roll in the millet flour and bake for 25 minutes.

Mustard sauce

Good for: Rotation Diet, Day 4

Serves 4

2 tbsp butter

3 tbsp tapioca flour

½ cup sheep's milk

1 tsp ground mustard

1 tbsp cider vinegar (optional)

sea salt

Melt the butter in a saucepan over gentle heat and stir in the flour to make a roux. Cook for 2 to 3 minutes, allowing it to bubble but not to change color. Remove from the heat and gradually stir in the milk. Return to the heat, add the mustard, vinegar, and salt, and stir until the sauce thickens.

Mayonnaise

Good for: Elimination Diet, Day 15

Serves 4

2 quail's egg yolks

1 whole quail's egg

1 tbsp lemon juice

½ tsp ground mustard

pinch white pepper

sea salt

1 cup walnut oil, olive oil, or mixture

Keep all the ingredients at room temperature. Place the eggs, lemon juice, and seasoning in a blender and mix for a few seconds. Turn on to maximum speed and slowly pour in the oil until it thickens.

Tofu mayonnaise

Good for: Elimination Diet, Day 25; Rotation Diet, Day 3

Serves 4

1 cup silken tofu

1 clove garlic, crushed (optional) (not for Day 3)

2 tbsp safflower or sunfower seed oil

2 tbsp cider vinegar (or wine vinigar for Day 3)

pinch of white pepper (not for Day 3)

sea salt to taste

Place all the ingredients in a blender and mix until smooth.

Egg mayonnaise

Good for: Rotation Diet, Day 3

Serves 4

2 egg yolks at room temperature

2 tbsp wine vinegar

½ tsp sea salt

1 cup safflower oil at room temperature

Place all the ingredients in a blender except for the oil, and blend for 1 minute. Remove the top from the blender, turn on to top speed, and add the oil a few drops at a time until the mixture thickens.

Ginger syrup

Good for: Elimination Diet, Day 18

Serves 4

½ cup water

1 tsp grated ginger

2 cups white grape juice

Bring the water to a boil and add the ginger. Cook for 2 to 3 minutes and add to the grape juice. Continue cooking until the liquid is reduced by half. Strain and use hot or cold.

Tomato sauce

Good for: Elimination Diet, Day 19

Serves 4

2¼ cups tomatoes, skinned, seeded, and cut into chunks

2 ribs celery, chopped

1 clove garlic, crushed

4 spring onions, chopped

1 tbsp tomato purée

1 tbsp fresh basil, chopped

sea salt

2 tbsp sunflower/safflower oil

Gently cook the vegetables until soft. Add the tomato purée, basil, and seasoning and cook for another minute. Stir in the oil before serving but do not heat.

Redcurrant sauce

Good for: Preliminary Diet

Serves 4

2¼ cups redcurrants

1 cup mineral water

1 tbsp fruit sugar, honey or maple syrup

2 tsp sago or tapioca flour

Place the redcurrants in a saucepan with the water. Bring to a boil and simmer until cooked. Add the sugar and thicken with the sago/tapioca flour mixed with a little cold water.

Horseradish sauce

Good for: Rotation Diet, Day 4

Serves 4

1 small dessert apple, peeled and cored
1 cup turnip, diced
1 tsp ground lemongrass
½ tsp ground mustard seed
sea salt
2 tsp tapioca flour, for thickening
½ cup fresh horseradish, grated

Cook the apple and turnip in a little water until tender. Cool slightly and purée in a blender with the seasonings. Return to the saucepan, reheat, and use a little tapioca flour to thicken. Stir in the grated horseradish and serve.

SALADS AND DRESSINGS

French dressing

Good for: Elimination Diet, Day 11

Serves 4

juice of 2 lemons
½ cup cold pressed virgin olive oil/walnut oil
1 tsp ground mustard
1 clove garlic, crushed
1 tsp fresh mint, chopped
½ tsp sea salt

Combine all the ingredients in a jar and shake well.

Salad dressing

Good for: Rotation Diet, Day 1

Serves 4

juice of 2 lemons

¼ cup oil (wheat germ oil and/or sesame seed oil)

1 tbsp tahini (optional)

½ tsp sea salt, black pepper

Combine all the ingredients in a jar and shake well.

Fresh green salad

Good for: Rotation Diet, Day 4

Serves 4

bok choy

watercress

shredded cabbage

sorrel leaves

Mix together any or all of the leaves and served with salad dressing.

Fresh winter salad

Good for: Rotation Diet, Day 4

Serves 4

grated raw rutabaga

kohlrabi

turnips

sliced radishes

water chestnuts

shredded white cabbage

red dessert apple, cut into segments

Mix together the ingredients and serve with a dressing or mustard sauce.

Fennel and bean sprout salad

Good for: Preliminary Diet; Elimination Diet, Day 25

Serves 4

1 large fennel, thinly sliced

2¼ cups bean sprouts

½ cucumber, sliced

1 zucchini, diced

1¼ cups seedless green grapes

1 nectarine, cut into segments

4 Chinese leaves, shredded

Arrange the ingredients on a bed of shredded Chinese leaves and serve with fresh mayonnaise or salad dressing, which may be made with cider vinegar.

Arame with sesame seeds

Good for: Preliminary Diet; Elimination Diet, Day 16

Serves 4

5 ounces dried and shredded arame

1 carrot, cut into matchsticks

¼ cup sesame seeds

Rinse the arame seaweed and place in a pan with enough cold water to cover and leave to soak for 10 minutes. Add the carrot and bring to a boil and simmer for 30 minutes until all the water has been absorbed. Turn into a serving dish. Sprinkle the sesame seeds on the top.

Melon, cucumber, and strawberry salad

Good for: Elimination Diet, Day 10

Serves 4

1 small lettuce, shredded

1 honeydew melon, cut into cubes

½ cucumber, cut in half and sliced

1¼ cups strawberries, sliced

pumpkin seeds

cold pressed olive oil

sprigs of fresh mint for garnishing

Place the shredded lettuce on a serving dish and arrange the other ingredients on top. Sprinkle with oil and garnish with mint.

Egg and pasta salad

Good for: Elimination Diet, Day 11

Serves 4

9 ounces buckwheat spirals

2 tsp olive oil

1 cup celery root, cut into strips and blanched

3 ribs celery, sliced

1 cup asparagus tips

½ cup walnuts

6 to 8 quail eggs, hard boiled and cut in half

1 tbsp dill, for garnishing

Cook the buckwheat in boiling water until al dente adding a little oil to the water to prevent sticking. Drain and allow to cool on a serving dish. Add the celery root, celery, asparagus tips, and walnuts, and arrange the eggs on the top. Pour over a little French dressing and garnish with dill.

Coleslaw

Good for: Elimination Diet, Day 15

Serves 4

2 red apples, cored and diced

1 tbsp lemon juice

1 small white cabbage, shredded

4 cups grated carrot

2 ribs celery, sliced

1 tbsp chopped chives

½ cup raisins

2 tbsp mayonnaise

chopped fresh parsley for garnishing

Toss the apple in lemon juice to prevent browning. Mix together all the dry ingredients, stir in the mayonnaise, and sprinkle with parsley.

Rice, barley, and bean sprout salad

Good for: Elimination Diet, Day 17

Serves 4

¾ cup cooked rice

¼ cup cooked pot barley

1 cup green beans, sliced and cooked

1 cup garden peas, cooked

1 cup bean sprouts

2 spring onions, chopped (optional)

salad dressing

4 heads of Belgian endive or 1 bunch of watercress for garnishing

Allow the cooked grains and vegetables to cool. Mix in with the remaining ingredients and pour over the salad dressing. Place in the center of a serving dish and arrange endive or watercress around the edge.

Prawn, avocado, and fennel salad with buckwheat pasta

Good for: Elimination Diet, Day 18

Serves 4

8 ounces buckwheat pasta

salad leaves

12 ounces peeled prawns

2 ripe avocados, sliced

1 bulb fennel, sliced

salad dressing (see page 198)

1 tsp dill

sprigs of thyme for garnishing

6 to 8 black olives for garnishing

Cook the pasta until al dente. Drain and allow to cool. Arrange the salad leaves on a serving dish and place the prawns, avocado pears, fennel, and buckwheat pasta on top. Spoon over the salad dressing, sprinkle with dill, and garnish with sprigs of thyme and black olives.

Couscous salad

Good for: Elimination Diet, Day 27

Serves 4

1 cup couscous

2½ cups boiling water

2 tomatoes, skinned and diced

1 small green pepper, deseeded and diced

2 spring onions, finely sliced

juice of 1 lemon

freshly chopped basil or mint

sea salt and black pepper

Rinse the couscous in a fine mesh strainer. Place in a bowl and pour on the hot water. Allow to stand for 15 minutes until the water has been absorbed. When cool, mix with the vegetables, herbs, and seasoning.

Greek salad

Good for: Elimination Diet, Day 20

Serves 4

1 small head of romaine lettuce

2 heads of Belgian endive

4 tomatoes, halved and sliced

½ cucumber, diced lengthways

1 small red pepper

1 small green pepper

¾ cup pitted black olives

1¼ cups Feta cheese, cut into cubes

French dressing (see page 197)

1 tsp oregano, for garnishing

Bunch the lettuce leaves together and cut into thin strips with a sharp knife. Place on the bottom of a serving dish and arrange the other ingredients on top. Spoon over the dressing and sprinkle with oregano.

Orange and fennel salad

Good for: Rotation Diet, Day 1

Serves 4

4 heads of fennel, sliced

2 large oranges, peeled and divided into segments

1 tbsp sprouted fennel seeds (optional)

2 to 3 sprigs of fennel leaf, for garnishing

salad dressing

Mix together all the ingredients and pour over the dressing.

Avocado sweet and sour salad

Good for: Elimination Diet, Day 23

Serves 4

FOR THE DRESSING

juice of 1 lemon

2 tbsp sweet almond oil

ground ginger

salt and black pepper

julienne strips of orange peel for garnishing

2 avocados, cut into chunks

lemon juice

4 cups carrots, finely shredded

4 cups mung bean sprouts

juice of 2 oranges

2 oranges divided into segments

⅓ cup organic golden raisins

Make the dressing by mixing together all the ingredients. Sprinkle the avocado with lemon juice to stop browning. Mix together all the salad items in a salad bowl and pour over the dressing.

Cucumber, avocado, and asparagus salad

Good for: Rotation Diet, Day 2

Serves 4

2 avocados

1 cup asparagus tips

1 cucumber, cut into chunks

paprika

sprig of mint, for garnishing

Cook the asparagus tips in water until just tender. Drain and cool. Halve the avocados, removing the skin and pit. Mix with the cucumber and asparagus and sprinkle with paprika. Garnish with mint.

Mixed grain salad

Good for: Rotation Diet, Day 1

Serves 4

½ cup cooked wheat barley or rye grains

½ cup cooked millet

⅔ cup cashew nuts, roughly chopped

sprouted seeds, e.g., dill, celery, aniseed

2 ribs celery, diced

1 cup grated carrot

salad dressing

1 tbsp sesame seeds for garnishing

freshly chopped parsley for garnishing

Mix together all the ingredients, keeping the sesame seeds and parsley for garnishing. Pour over the salad dressing. The grains may also be used, sprouted.

Green bean salad

Good for: Rotation Diet, Day 3

Serves 4

3 cups green beans, cut in halves

sea salt

cold-pressed safflower or sunflower seed oil

1 hard boiled egg, grated

3½ cups alfalfa sprouts

Place the beans in a saucepan with a pinch of salt and enough boiling water to cover. Cook for 7 to 10 minutes until tender. Drain well and toss in a little oil. Place in the middle of a serving dish and sprinkle with the sieved egg. Place the alfalfa sprouts around the edge of the dish. The egg may be replaced with chopped walnuts.

Seafood salad

Good for: Rotation Diet, Day 1

Serves 4

8 ounces pasta spirals, wheat, rye, barley, or millet

1 lb mussels

8 to 10 baby squid tentacles, cut from the bodies

8 ounces peeled prawns

salad dressing

2 tbsp freshly chopped parsley for garnishing

To cook the pasta, fill a large saucepan with water and bring to a boil. Add the pasta and a pinch of salt. Cook until just tender, for 8 to 10 minutes according to the type of pasta used.

To prepare the mussels, pull off the beards and thoroughly wash and scrub the shells. Place in a shallow pan and cover with boiling water. Cook for 5 minutes, shaking the pan now and then. Remove the mussels as soon as the shells open, and discard any that do not open.

Place the squid pieces in the mussel water and cook for 15 minutes until tender. Add the prawns and cook for another 5 minutes. Drain and allow to cool. Cut the squid into rings and mix with the mussels, prawns, and cooked pasta.

Arrange on a serving dish, pour over the salad dressing, and sprinkle with chopped parsley.

Cherry and almond salad

Good for: Rotation Diet, Day 3

Serves 4

1½ cups black cherries

1 nectarine

1 small head of romaine lettuce

1 cup almonds, blanched

cold-pressed, unrefined safflower or sunflower seed oil

Wash and pit the cherries, reserving a few with stalks for garnishing. Wash the nectarine and cut into small segments. Arrange the lettuce leaves around the edge of the plate and pile the fruit on top with the almonds. Sprinkle with oil and garnish with the whole cherries.

Pear and watercress salad

Good for: Rotation Diet, Day 4

Serves 4

4 ripe pears

1 bunch watercress, washed

2 tbsp cold-pressed walnut oil

½ tsp ground mustard seeds

Peel and quarter the pears and quickly immerse them in salt water to prevent browning. Arrange in a serving bowl with the watercress, spoon over the oil, and sprinkle with mustard seed.

BREADS, CAKES, AND BISCUITS

Barley scone bread

Good for: Elimination Diet, Days 10 & 12

Serves 4

1¾ cups barley flour

¼ cup olive oil

⅔ cup cashew nuts, chopped (optional)

1 tsp baking soda

5 tbsp water

sea salt

Preheat the oven to 325°F.

Mix together all the ingredients and make into a large scone. Divide into 4 pieces. Bake for 20 to 25 minutes.

Cornbread

Good for: Elimination Diet, Day 16; Rotation Diet, Day 2

Serves 4

1¼ cups corn flour

⅓ cup cooked squash or pumpkin

1 tsp cream of tartar

½ tsp baking soda

¼ cup olive oil

1 cup water

2½ tsp honey (fruit sugar for Day 2)

Preheat the oven to 300°F and line a loaf tin with wax paper.

Mix together all the ingredients and bake for 40 to 45 minutes until firm.

Rice bread

Good for: Preliminary Diet

Serves 4

1¼ cups rice flakes

1¾ cups mineral water

1 cup pea or lentil flour

¾ cup almonds or brazil nuts, ground

1¼ cups kohlrabi, grated or turnip

2 tbsp sesame seed oil or olive oil

1 tbsp tapioca flour or arrowroot

1 tsp cream of tartar

½ tsp baking soda

½ tsp sea salt

Preheat the oven to 300°F and line a loaf tin with wax paper.

Pour the water onto the rice flakes to soften. Mix all the ingredients, transfer to the loaf tin, and bake for 1 hour until firm.

Raisin bun loaf

Good for: Preliminary Diet; Rotation Diet, Day 3

Serves 4

For the Preliminary Diet, follow the recipe for rice bread and add 1 cup raisins.

For Rotation Diet, follow the recipe for rice and sago bread and add 1 cup raisins.

Rice and sago bread

Good for: Preliminary Diet; Rotation Diet, Day 3

Serves 4

¾ cup sago pearls

1½ cups mineral water

¾ cup rice flour

⅓ cup lentil flour

1 tsp cream of tartar

½ tsp baking soda

Preheat the oven to 300°F and line a loaf tin with wax paper.

Pour the water onto the sago and leave to soak for 30 minutes to soften. Mix with the remaining ingredients, transfer to the loaf tin, and bake for 45 minutes.

Soda bread

Good for: Rotation Diet, Day 1

Serves 4

3 cups permissible flour

1 tsp baking soda

½ tsp salt (optional)

1 cup water or nut milk

Preheat the oven to 350°F.

Mix together all the ingredients and form into a firm dough. Shape into a flat round loaf, cut a deep cross on top, and bake for 40 minutes until firm.

Rye bread

Good for: Elimination Diet, Day 20; Rotation Diet, Day 1

Serves 4

3 tbsp fresh yeast

1 tsp raw cane molasses sugar

1 cup warm water

½ tsp salt

3 cups rye flour

1 tsp caraway seeds

Mix the yeast with the sugar and pour on half the water. Leave for 5 to 10 minutes for it to froth. Add the salt to the flour and pour in the yeast mixture. Add the caraway seeds and the remaining water and mix to a dough. Knead for 5 to 10 minutes and then leave covered in a warm place until it has doubled in size. Knock back and knead again for 2 to 3 minutes. Form into two round loaves and place on a well-greased baking tray. Cover and leave for 30 minutes until well risen. Preheat the oven to 400°F.

Bake the loaves for 10 minutes at 400°F, then reduce the oven setting to 350°F and bake for another 25 minutes.

Russian-style rye bread can be made with just rye flour, water, and salt. Whole-meal wheat or spelt wheat bread can be made following the above recipe but substituting the wheat flour for rye and reducing the quantity of yeast to 5 tsp. Omit the caraway seeds and use cashew nuts or a few wheat flakes instead. Sprinkle with sesame seeds, poppyseeds, or wheat flakes.

Sprouted grain bread

Good for: Elimination Diet, Day 27; Rotation Diet, Day 1

Serves 4

3 cups organic wheat grains

filtered water for sprouting

sea salt

Rinse the grains and leave to soak for 15 hours. Drain off the water and leave to sprout for two to three days until the grains have developed 1" sprouts, rinsing morning and evening.

Preheat the oven to 275°F. Place the grains in a meat mincer and grind the sprouts to a fine texture. Add the salt and place in a well-oiled loaf tin and bake for 4 to 5 hours, until the bread leaves the sides of the tin.

Buckwheat chapatis

Good for: Elimination Diet, Day 23; Rotation Diet, Day 4

Serves 4

1¼ cups buckwheat flour

water

Mix the flour with enough water to make a firm dough. Break off small pieces and roll out into very thin rounds. Cook in a dry frying pan until brown, then grill under a hot grill until they puff up.

Pita bread

Good for: Rotation Diet, Day 1

Serves 4

5 tsp fresh or dried yeast

1 tsp unrefined molasses sugar

1 cup warm water

1 tsp salt

3 cups organic strong whole wheat flour or barley flour

FOR THE HERB AND SESAME TOPPING (OPTIONAL)

sesame seed oil

2½ tbsp chopped fresh parsley or cilantro

2½ tbsp sesame seeds

Mix the yeast, sugar, and water and leave in a warm place for 5 to 10 minutes until frothy. Mix the salt with the flour and combine with the yeast liquid to form a soft dough. Knead for 10 minutes. Place in a large, oiled polythene bag and leave in a warm place until doubled in size. Preheat the oven to 425°F.

On a floured board, knead the dough for a minute and divide into eight portions. Knead each portion into a small ball and roll out into an oval shape and lay these onto several oiled baking trays. Cover with oiled polythene and leave to rest for 30 minutes.

Brush with sesame seed oil and sprinkle with herbs and sesame seeds. Bake for 8 minutes until risen and puffed.

Celebration carrot cake

Good for: Elimination Diet, Day 28

Serves 4

1¼ cups wholemeal flour

2½ cups shredded carrot

1 cup crushed pineapple and juice

⅔ cup coconut

⅔ cup walnuts, chopped

3 eggs, beaten

1 tsp cream of tartar

½ tsp baking soda

½ cup butter or oil

2 tsp cinnamon

2 tsp natural vanilla essence

Preheat the oven to 300°F and line and grease a cake tin.

Mix together all the ingredients, transfer to the cake tin, and bake for 40 minutes.

Pineapple upside-down cake

Good for: Rotation Diet, Day 2

Serves 4

1 pineapple, sliced

1½ cups corn flour

1½ cups corn starch

½ cup corn syrup

½ cup olive oil

2 cups water

1 tsp baking soda

Preheat the oven to 325°F. Put the sliced pineapple into the bottom of a well-oiled ovenproof dish. Mix together the other ingredients and pour onto the fruit. Cook for 45 minutes until firm.

Apple and hazelnut muffins

Good for: Rotation Diet, Day 4

Serves 4

¾ cups hazelnuts, skinned and chopped

1¼ cups sweet potato, baked, skinned and cooled

1 cup buckwheat flour

1 large or 2 small eating apples, peeled and chopped

½ cup butter

1 tbsp maple syrup (optional)

1 tsp allspice

Preheat the oven to 300°F and grease 9 muffin tins.

To remove the skins from the hazelnuts, place in a grill pan and grill lightly for 2 to 3 minutes, watching carefully. Rub the nuts between two sheets of kitchen paper or in a clean tea towel and the skins will flake off.

Mix together all the ingredients and put into the muffin tins. Bake for 15 to 20 minutes.

Barley and cashew nut scones

Good for: Rotation Diet, Day 1

Serves 4

1½ cups barley flour

1 tsp baking soda

1 cup cashew nuts, ground or chopped

¼ cup sesame seed oil

1 tsp sugar (optional)

1 cup water

Preheat the oven to 325°F.

Mix together the ingredients and form into a firm dough. Cut into individual scones with a pastry cutter or make one large scone, cutting a cross on the top. Bake for 10 to 15 minutes, according to size.

Green banana and oatmeal scones

Good for: Rotation Diet, Day 2

Serves 4

1¼ cups green banana flour

1¼ cups fine oatmeal

2 tbsp fruit sugar (fructose)

1 tsp baking soda

2 tbsp olive oil

1 cup nut milk or water

Preheat the oven to 325°F.

Place the dry ingredients in a large bowl and rub in the oil. Add sufficient nut milk/water to form a firm dough. Roll out to about ¾" thickness and cut into rounds with a 2" cutter. Bake for 10 to 15 minutes.

Buckwheat and chestnut dropped scones

Good for: Rotation Diet, Day 4

Serves 4

1⅓ cups buckwheat flour

1⅓ cups chestnut flour

2½ cups water

Mix together the flours and the water. Drop in spoonfuls onto a hot griddle, dropping from the point of the spoon to keep the scone in good shape. Allow 1 tablespoon for each scone. When bubbles appear and the scone is just beginning to brown on the underside, turn with a flat spatula and cook on the other side.

Delicious served with apple and pear spread; strawberry or raspberry sugarless jams; or with yogurt, pecan nuts, and maple syrup.

Carrot and fig slice

Good for: Rotation Diet, Day 1

Serves 4

1 cup dried figs

1¼ cups whole wheat flour

3½ cups grated carrot

⅓ cup sesame seed oil

½ tsp aniseed

Preheat the oven to 325°F and grease or line an 8" baking pan.

Place the figs in a saucepan, cover with water and cook for 20 minutes. Drain and blend to a purée. Mix the purée with the rest of the ingredients, spoon into the baking pan, and bake for 1 hour. Allow to cool before turning out.

Cherry and coconut slices

Good for: Rotation Diet, Day 3

Serves 4

½ cup rice flakes soaked in 1 cup water

3–5 tbsp honey

¼ cup almond oil

2 eggs beaten

⅓ cup desiccated coconut

⅓ cup dried cherries

Preheat the oven to 325°F and oil or line a 8" baking tin.

Mix together all the ingredients and turn into the baking tin. Bake for 25 to 30 minutes until firm to the touch.

Orange and cashew nut crunchies

Good for: Rotation Diet, Day 1

Serves 4

¼ cup sesame seed oil

⅔ cup raw cane sugar or barley malt

1½ cups whole-meal flour

¾ cup ground cashew nuts

grated zest of 1 orange

Preheat the oven to 350°F and grease a Swiss roll tin.

Warm the oil and cane sugar/barley malt in a saucepan for 2 to 3 minutes. Mix with the remaining ingredients and spoon into the Swiss roll tin and bake for 15 to 20 minutes. Allow to cool before cutting into fingers or squares.

Chocolate hazelnut biscuits

Good for: Elimination Diet, Day 26

Serves 4

1½ cups wheat flour or fine oatmeal

1 tsp cream of tartar

½ tsp bicarbonate of soda

⅔ cup fruit sugar

½ cup cocoa powder

1 tsp natural vanilla essence

½ cup chopped hazelnuts for decoration

Preheat the oven to 300°F and line a baking sheet with greaseproof paper.

Mix together all the ingredients and divide into pieces the size of a walnut. Place on the lined baking sheet and flatten with a fork dipped in cold water. Decorate with nuts. Bake for 25 to 20 minutes. Allow to cool before lifting on to a wire rack.

If using oatmeal, replace 1 tbsp with 1 tbsp tapioca or arrowroot flour.

Brazil nut cookies

Good for: Rotation Diet, Day 2

Serves 4

1¼ cups fine oatmeal flour

½ cup rolled oats

1 cup Brazil nuts, finely chopped

⅓ cup fruit sugar

¼ cup olive oil

water to mix

1 tsp arrowroot or cornflour

Preheat the oven to 325°F and grease a baking sheet.

Place all the dry ingredients in a large mixing bowl and rub in the oil. Add sufficient water to make a firm dough. Roll out on a surface dusted with arrowroot or corn flour and cut with a biscuit cutter. Place on the baking sheet and cook for 10 to 15 minutes until light golden in color.

DESSERTS

Fig and lime sorbet

Good for: Rotation Diet, Day 1

Serves 4

6 fresh figs

juice of 2 limes

cane sugar to taste

2 level tsp agar

FOR THE DECORATION

1 fresh fig, sliced thinly

julienne strips of lime

Wash and cut the figs into quarters and place in a saucepan. Bring to a boil, cover, and gently cook for 5 minutes.

Allow to cool a little and blend, adding the lime juice, sugar, and agar dissolved in a little hot water. Spoon into a freezer container and freeze for 1 to 2 hours until almost frozen. Return to the blender and whip until light and fluffy. Return to the freezer until firm.

Scoop the ice cream to serve and decorate.

Blood oranges with cranberries

Good for: Rotation Diet, Day 1

Serves 4

4 blood oranges

zest of 1 orange

1¾ cups cranberries

1 tbsp raw cane sugar

Cut the oranges into segments and the zest into julienne strips. Cook the cranberries for 2 to 3 minutes with the julienne strips and sugar. Allow to cool and then mix with the oranges. (May be enhanced with a little cinnamon from Day 2).

Chicory coffee ice cream

Good for: Rotation Diet, Day 3

Serves 4

2 eggs or soy egg substitute

⅓ cup honey

¼ cup almond oil

2½ cups soy milk

2 tsp instant chicory coffee granules

¾ cup ground almonds, for the topping

Beat the eggs and blend with the remaining ingredients. Place in a shallow freezing tray and freeze until just beginning to set. Take out and whisk until light and fluffy. Return to the freezer. Serve with a topping of ground almonds.

Pistachio nut semolina with lime

Good for: Rotation Diet, Day 1

Serves 4

2 cups cashew nut milk

zest of 1 lime and juice of 2 limes

2½ cups raw cane sugar

2½ cups semolina

¾ cup unsalted pistachio nuts, chopped

Bring the cashew nut milk to a boil and add the zest of lime cut into julienne strips. Add the sugar and sprinkle in the semolina, stirring briskly until the mixture thickens. Cool and stir in the lime juice and chopped pistachio nuts, keeping a few for decoration.

Grilled pineapple with macadamia nuts

Good for: Rotation Diet, Day 2

Serves 4

1 large pineapple
1 tbsp fruit sugar
⅔ cup macadamia nuts, sliced

Using a serrated knife, trim off about ½" from each end of the pineapple, saving some of the leaves. Cut into quarters lengthways and carefully trim away the core, then cut along the base of each quarter so the flesh is separated from the skin. Cut the flesh in half lengthways and then into four crossways to give bite-sized portions.

Sprinkle each quarter with fruit sugar and place under a grill until just beginning to caramelise. Decorate with macadamia nuts and serve.

Fruit crêpes

Good for: Rotation Diet, Day 2

Serves 4

1 cup fine oatmeal, corn, or quinoa flour
½ cup corn starch or green banana flour
1 tsp fruit sugar
1 cup nut milk or water

Place all the dry ingredients in a bowl and add half the liquid. Beat well to form a smooth, thick batter. Gradually add the remaining liquid to produce a pouring consistency. Spoon 2 to 3 tbsp of the mixture on to a hot griddle and cook on both sides until just golden. Serve hot with a fruit filling of your choice.

Damson (Asian plum) syllabub

Good for: Rotation Diet, Day 3

Serves 4

2½ cups damsons or plums

¼ cup unrefined beet sugar or honey

½ cup water

1 tbsp sago flour

2 egg whites

Wash the damsons/plums. Place the sugar in a saucepan with the water and stir over a gentle heat, until dissolved. Add the damsons, cover and simmer until soft. Mix the sago with a little cold water and stir into the damsons. Sieve into a large bowl, discard the pits, and allow to cool.

Beat the egg whites until white and fluffy but not dry. Gently fold into the damsons and spoon the mixture into individual glass bowls.

Tapioca milk pudding

Good for: Rotation Diet, Day 4

Serves 4

⅓ cup tapioca flakes

4¼ cups sheep's milk

1 tbsp maple syrup

pat of butter, sugarless jam, or stewed or fresh fruit (optional)

Soak the tapioca in the milk for 1 hour. Gently simmer the tapioca in the milk, stirring from time to time, until cooked. Serve with a pat of butter, a spoonful of sugarless jam, or with stewed or fresh fruit.

Apricot and almond flan

Good for: Rotation Diet, Day 3

Serves 4

FOR THE RICE PASTRY

1¼ cups rice flour

⅓ cup soy flour

½ cup almond oil

½ cup water

FOR THE APRICOT FILLING

3⅓ cups apricots

1 cup water

1 to 2 tbsp honey (optional)

¾ cup ground almonds

⅔ cup flaked or chopped almonds

Preheat the oven to 300°F and oil a flan dish very thoroughly.

For the pastry, mix together all the ingredients. This dough does not roll easily, so it is better to pat down evenly into the flan dish.

For the filling, take half the apricots and place in a saucepan with the water and honey, if using. Bring to a boil and simmer until cooked. When cool, blend to a purée.

Make a layer of the ground almonds on top of the pastry base. Cut the remaining raw apricots into halves or slices and arrange on top of the ground almonds. Pour over the apricot purée and decorate the flan with the flaked almonds. Bake for 35 minutes.

Steamed apple pudding

Good for: Rotation Diet, Day 4

Serves 4

1¼ cups sweet potato, baked, skinned and cooled

1 cup buckwheat flour

2 large eating apples, peeled and chopped

½ cup butter

1 tbsp concentrated apple juice

1 tsp ground cloves

Mix together all the ingredients. Butter a 1 quart bowl and pour in the mixture. Cover with a double layer of wax paper. Steam in a saucepan of simmering water for 1 hour or for 30 minutes in a pressure cooker.

Bramble mousse

Good for: Rotation Diet, Day 4

Serves 4

4½ cups blackberries

½ cup water

3 tbsp concentrated apple juice

3 tbsp cold water

3 tsp powdered gelatin

½ cup double cream

Thoroughly wash the blackberries and place in a saucepan with the water and the apple concentrate to sweeten. Bring to a boil and simmer for 5 minutes until soft.

Put the cold water in a bowl, sprinkle on the gelatin, and allow to stand for 3 minutes. Stir into the fruit and rub through a sieve to remove the seeds and to make a purée. Allow to cool. Whisk the cream until it forms soft peaks, and fold into the purée before it sets.

Pears in raspberry sauce

Good for: Rotation Diet, Day 4

Serves 4

2 cups water

4 firm but ripe pears, peeled

½ cup raspberries

2 to 3 tbsp maple syrup

Put the water in a shallow pan and bring to a boil. Add the pears and poach for 10 to 12 minutes until they look slightly translucent but still firm. Lift out into a serving dish and cook the raspberries in the poaching water for 2 to 3 minutes. Press the raspberries through a sieve to remove the seeds, add the maple syrup to the juice, and spoon this over the pears. May be served with crème fraîche or live yogurt.

DRINKS AND DAIRY SUBSTITUTES

Lemon and orange barley water

Good for: Rotation Diet, Day 1

Serves 4

¼ cup pot barley

4¼ cups water

2 tbsp barley malt

2 oranges

1 lemon

Place the barley in a saucepan with the water. Bring to a boil and simmer for 1 hour. Stir in the barley malt and leave to cool.

Wash the fruit and grate the zest into a jug. Cut away the pith and discard. Thinly slice the flesh and add to the zest. Strain the barley water and pour into the jug with the fruit.

Lemon and elderflower cordial

Good for: Rotation Diet, Day 1

Serves 4

grated zest of 1 lemon and juice of 2 lemons
10 heads of freshly gathered elderflowers or 1 ounce dried elderflowers
2 tbsp raw cane sugar
4¼ cups boiling water

Place the lemon zest, elderflowers, and sugar in a saucepan and pour on a boiling water. Leave for 10 to 20 minutes and strain off the juice. Add the fresh lemon juice and serve chilled with slices of lemon. Dilute to taste.

Elderberry punch

Good for: Rotation Diet, Day 1

Serves 4

2 lbs elderberries
2 cups water
zest and juice of 2 lemons
4¼ cups orange juice
2 cups green leaf tea, strained
2 tbsp grenadine (optional)
½ tbsp cane sugar or to taste
2 oranges, sliced

Place the elderberries in a large saucepan with the water and lemon zest and bring to a boil. Simmer for 10 minutes and then strain off the pulp. Pour the elderberry juice back into the saucepan and add the orange juice, lemon juice, tea, and grenadine, if using. Add sugar to taste. Bring to a boil and then simmer for 10 minutes. Place slices of orange in a jug and pour on the punch. Serve hot.

This may be served chilled or as a hot punch with 2 sticks of cinnamon and 2 to 3 sprigs of thyme (from Rotation Diet, Day 2).

Strawberry yogurt crush

Good for: Rotation Diet, Day 4

Serves 4

1 cup strawberries, washed and hulled

1 cup live sheep's yogurt

2½ tbsp maple syrup

1 cup water or cold lemongrass tea

ice cubes (optional)

Blend all the ingredients until smooth, adding the ice cubes (if using) a second or two at the end.

Rose hip cordial

Good for: Rotation Diet, Day 4

Serves 4

Gather well-ripened rose hips from the wild in the early autumn or from garden roses throughout the summer. Wash thoroughly and cut in half, lengthways. Place in a saucepan with enough water to float them and bring to a boil. Simmer gently for 30 minutes and strain. Sweeten with maple, concentrated apple/pear juice, or rice syrup, according to taste, and use in drinks. May be mixed with blackberries or raspberries.

Banana milk shake

Good for: Rotation Diet, Day 2

Serves 4

1 peeled banana

2 cups nut or oat milk

Place the ingredients in a blender and mix until smooth. Serve immediately.

Tiger nut milk

Good for: Preliminary Diet; Elimination Diet, Day 7; Rotation Diet,
Day 2

Serves 4

1 cup tiger nuts washed and soaked overnight
4¼ cups mineral water

Rinse the tiger nuts. Blend with the water and strain off the pulp. Use poured over cereal, and keep or freeze the pulp to use in recipes.

Oat milk

Good for: Elimination Diet, Day 16; Rotation Diet, Day 2

Serves 4

½ cup oatmeal or flakes
4¼ cups water
1 tsp fruit sugar (optional)
drop of natural vanilla essence (optional)

Place the oats in a large pan with the water and bring to a boil. Simmer for 10 minutes. Cool slightly, blend until smooth, and strain. Serve hot or cold, but it is a particularly delicious and warming drink served hot with a little sweetener.

Hemp seed milk

Good for: Rotation Diet, Day 2

Serves 4

½ cup hemp seeds, soaked for 48 hours
4¼ cups water

Place the seeds in a pan with the water and bring to a boil. Simmer for 15 to 20 minutes. Remove from the heat as soon as a yellow film starts to form on the surface. Leave to cool for a few minutes and then pour through a fine strainer or coffee filter. Serve chilled.

Rice milk

Good for: Preliminary Diet; Elimination Diet, Day 5; Rotation Diet,
    Day 3

Serves 4

¼ organic, short, whole-grain rice

4¼ cups mineral water

1 vanilla pod (optional)

1 to 2 tsp honey (optional)

1 tbsp safflower oil (optional)

Wash the grains and place in a saucepan with the water. Bring to
a boil with the vanilla pod and simmer gently for 20 minutes to
1 hour. Cool slightly and then mix in a blender. Pour through a
strainer and discard the pulp, or use in recipes. Add the honey, and
more water if necessary. Add the safflower oil when completely cool,
and keep refrigerated.

Cashew nut milk

Good for: Rotation Diet, Day 1

Serves 4

1 cup cashew nuts

4¼ cups water

1 tbsp barley malt (optional)

Grind the cashew nuts in a blender to a fine powder. Add some
of the water and all of the barley malt and blend until smooth,
gradually adding the remaining water. Keep chilled.

Almond milk

Good for: Preliminary Diet

Serves 4

1 cup blanched almonds

4¼ cups mineral water

1 to 2 tsp honey

pinch of cinnamon

Blend the almonds and some of the water for a good minute, until the mixture is very smooth. Add the honey, cinnamon, and remaining water, then strain and serve. Cashew nuts may also be used.

Walnut, pecan nut, and brazil nut milks can all be made in the same way.

Sunflower and sesame seed milk

Good for: Preliminary Diet

Serves 4

⅓ cup organic sunflower seeds

2 tbsp sesame seeds

2 cups mineral water

⅓ cup organic dried dates

Rinse the seeds and blend with some of the water. When smooth, add the dates and the remaining water, blend again, and serve. The fruit and seeds may be presoaked overnight.

Hot chocolate

Good for: Rotation Diet, Day 3

Serves 2

2½ cups rice or soy milk

2 tsp cocoa powder

2 tsp honey

Bring the milk to a boil and stir in the cocoa powder and honey.

Soy milk

Good for: Elimination Diet, Day 13; Rotation Diet, Day 3

Serves 4

2 cups organic soy beans

4¼ cups water

1 vanilla pod

1 tbsp safflower oil

1 to 2 tsp honey

Soak and sprout the soy beans for 4 to 5 days, rinsing twice a day. Place in a saucepan with the water and vanilla pod. Bring to a boil and then simmer gently until tender. Remove the vanilla pod and blend. Pour through a strainer, add the oil and honey to taste, and extra water if necessary. Grape juice can also be used as a sweetener.

Precooked soy flour may be used instead of beans, and the ingredients blended together.

Honey eggnog

Good for: Rotation Diet, Day 3

Serves 2

2½ cups rice milk (see page 234)

2 tsp honey

1 large free-range egg

pinch of nutmeg

Beat together the milk, honey, and egg and sprinkle with nutmeg. 1 tbsp of carob powder can be added.

Carrot and cashew nut spread

Good for: Rotation Diet, Day 1

Serves 4

¾ cup carrots, cooked and puréed

¾ cup cashew nuts, ground

1 tbsp fresh parsley, finely chopped

pinch of sea salt or 1 tsp barley miso

sesame oil (optional)

Mix together the ingredients, adding a little sesame oil if necessary.

Mushroom and tahini spread

Good for: Rotation Diet, Day 1

Serves 4

1¼ cups mushrooms, sliced

1 tbsp sesame oil

2 tbsp tahini

1 tbsp lemon juice

1 tsp barley miso

1 tbsp fresh parsley, finely chopped

Cook the mushrooms in the sesame seed oil until soft. Blend to a purée, and mix well with the remaining ingredients.

Brazil nut butter

Good for: Rotation Diet, Day 2

Serves 4

¾ cups Brazil nuts

virgin olive oil

Wash the nuts and leave to soak overnight. Rinse off the water and then blend, dropping the nuts one by one onto the rotary blades. Add a little virgin olive oil to make a smooth paste. Eat immediately or freeze.

Hemp seed butter

Good for: Rotation Diet, Day 2

Serves 4

¾ cup hemp seeds

virgin olive oil

sea salt

Follow the recipe for Brazil nut butter, but soak the hemp seeds for 48 hours before blending. The seeds may be lightly toasted using a dry frying pan and removing from the heat the moment they begin to pop.

Almond and sunflower seed butters

Good for: Rotation Diet, Day 3

Serves 4

Presoak the almonds or sunflower seeds overnight. Rinse and then blend, dropping a few nuts or seeds at a time onto the rotary blades. Add a pinch of salt to taste and a little of the corresponding coldpressed oil to make a paste. Use the same day or freeze.

Nut and seed butters

Good for: Preliminary Diet

Serves 4

Use any type of raw nut (except peanuts) or seed (presoaking overnight will make them sweeter and more digestible) and follow the method for almond and sunflower seed butters.

Hazelnut, walnut, or pecan nut butter

Good for: Rotation Diet, Day 4

Serves 4

¾ cup hazelnuts

¾ cup walnuts or pecan nuts

1 tbsp walnut oil

sea salt

Use raw nuts and presoak if you wish. Grind in a blender, dropping a few nuts at a time onto the rotary blades. Add a pinch of salt to taste and a little of the corresponding nut oil to make a paste. Spoon into a screwtop jar and store in the refrigerator.

Hedgerow jam

Good for: Preliminary Diet

Makes approximately 6 x 1 cup pots

6 cups blackberries

2 cups elderberries

2 cups rose hips

½ cup sloes

2 cups mineral water

1 cup pear juice

2 tbsp arrowroot or tapioca flour

Wash the fruit thoroughly and then stew in the water until soft. Pour through a sieve, stir in the pear juice to sweeten, and thicken with arrowroot or tapioca flour. Keep refrigerated or freeze in small portions.

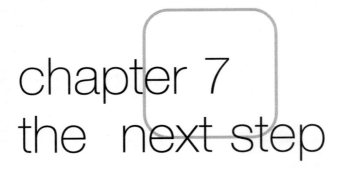

chapter 7
the next step

You can also help your body recover by strengthening your immune system. A strong immune system will be able to fight off viruses, bacteria, and other organisms and protect you from radiation, chemical pollution, and all other toxic and poisonous substances far more effectively. This, in turn, will give your body more of a chance to rebalance, thus making any reactions less and less severe.

Deficiencies in vitamins or minerals can have a debilitating effect on the immune system, so it is important to eat good, nourishing food. Additional food supplements may also be necessary, especially when many foods need to be eliminated or when the nutrients in the foods are not being absorbed properly, which is often the case with allergy sufferers. However, it would be wise to consult a health practitioner before embarking on a program so you do not waste money buying supplements of poor quality or ones that may cause adverse reactions. He or she will also be able to advise you on quantities. Here are some supplements that may be prescribed and prove to be useful:

Digestive enzymes These can help break down undigested food components such as proteins. They consist of hydrochloric acid and pepsin, normally present in the stomach, and pancreatic enzymes normally present in the duodenum and small intestines. An alternative is to eat more raw food, as the enzymes in the food will not have been destroyed by cooking.

Probiotics

These are a way of recolonizing good bacteria that may have been destroyed by drugs or poor diet. If harmful bacteria are allowed to take over, it can lead to conditions such as candidiasis. However, care needs to be taken in choosing a good quality supplement that contains Lactobacillus acidophilus and Bifidobacterium, either separately or together. Capsules should be bought in vacuum-sealed bottles and, once opened, kept in the refrigerator.

Soluble fiber

This helps to speed up the transport of food through the intestines. The longer poorly digested food stays in the gut, the more likely it is to cause problems. Fiber also helps to clean the walls of the intestines. The best sources are oat bran, rice bran, pectin, and physillium husks.

Essential fatty acids (EFAs)

These are vital for the immune system, for the health and protection of the gastro-intestinal mucosa and the cell membranes throughout the body. The essential fatty acids are omega-3 (alpha linolenic acid) and omega-6 (linoleic acid). Flaxseed oil is one of the best and richest sources of omega-3. This is also present in soy bean, walnut, and wheat germ oils. Omega-6 EFAs are found in sesame seed oil, safflower, sunflower, corn, and evening primrose oil. These oils should be unrefined and cold pressed and kept refrigerated once opened, as oils can become rancid quite quickly and in this state they can affect the body adversely. Deficiency can result in stunted growth, hair loss, varicose veins, brittle nails, sexual immaturity, nervousness, and skin disorders—especially eczema and dandruff.

Minerals and Multivitamins

These may be necessary, as it is increasingly difficult to obtain all the necessary amounts from foods alone.

Antioxidants

These include vitamins A,C,E; selenium, zinc, L-Cysteine and L-Glutathione. Apart from being important nutrients, these vitamins and minerals protect cells against harmful free radicals.

A free radical is an atom or molecule with an unpaired electron. It can be extremely damaging because it attempts to pair its free electron with an electron from neighboring molecules and can then set up a chain reaction causing damage to further cells. This "latching on" process is called oxidation and can "rust" the body almost as it does metal. Free radicals form because people are being exposed to thousands of substances, alien to the human body, such as atmospheric pollution, radiation, pesticides, additives, tobacco, alcohol, hard physical exercise, and many forms of medicines. Unsaturated fats, which are found naturally in cell membranes, are particularly susceptible to free radical damage. The cell walls then become vulnerable to cancer, arteriosclerosis, arthritis, premature aging, and other diseases.

Vitamin C

This also has natural anti-inflammatory properties, and it is important for iron absorption and in the production of collagen, a protein necessary for the formation of connective tissue in the skin, ligaments, and bones. It also helps to control blood cholesterol levels and is an anti-stress factor. Deficiency may show itself in swollen gums, weakened enamel or dentine, sore joints, fatigue, lowered resistance to infection, nosebleeds, slow healing of wounds, and poor complexion.

Ginkgo biloba

This is an herb that is also a powerful antioxidant and a useful protector for the intestinal mucosa. It improves the blood circulation in the hands, legs, feet, and in the brain, thus improving memory and concentration.

The B vitamins

These are a group of vitamins that are essential for the release of energy from food and vital for the metabolism of proteins and fats. They help maintain good circulation and healthy skin, hair, and eyes. They contribute to the functioning of the brain and nervous system, to maintaining the correct balance of hormones in the body, and to increasing one's ability to deal with stress.

Magnesium This is needed for the metabolism of carbohydrates to release energy, for nerve impulse transmission and brain function and for normal muscle function, including that of the heart. Symptoms of deficiency may include apprehensiveness, muscle twitches, tremors, confusion and forgetfulness, sleeplessness, the formation of clots in the heart and brain; and may contribute to calcium deposits in the kidneys, blood vessels, and heart. Our soil and, hence, the vegetable levels, are low, so most of us could do with extra.

Iodine This aids in the development and functioning of the thyroid gland, being a chief constituent of thyroxin, a principle hormone, and is particularly important for children and the elderly. Iodine plays an important role in regulating the body's production of energy, and it stimulates the rate of metabolism, helping the body to burn off excess fat. Mentality, speech, and the condition of the hair, nails, and skin and teeth are dependent upon a well-functioning thyroid gland. Iodine is necessary for neutralizing certain toxic substances and for protecting the body from the harmful effects of radiation. It is found in seaweed or can be taken in the form of kelp powder or tablets. Some kelp tablets contain milk powder, whey, or lactose.

Zinc This is necessary for the production of a vast number of enzymes and hormones present in the body. This is also a mineral that has become very depleted in the soil. Stretch marks in the skin and white spots on the nails can be a sign of zinc deficiency. It may also produce an increase in fatigue, susceptibility to infection, and a decrease in mental alertness.

Other ways of strengthening the immune system

In addition to diet and nutrition, we need to look at other aspects of our lives in order to strengthen our immune system and receive the benefits of good health. This includes getting sufficient exercise, fresh air, and sunlight; our ability to relax; looking at our posture and breathing habits; and above all, the quality of our thoughts.

We owe it to ourselves to be well. If we are well, we have energy, vitality, and are a joy to be with. Health also gives us the ability to work and achieve our aims in life. Perhaps we think that by ignoring

---

Case study

Mary, age 49, was bothered by a lot of symptoms. She was overweight, had itching skin, tingling in her legs, weeping eyes, sensitivity to bright lights, hot flashes, palpitations, water retention, bloating, thrush, backache, pain in her muscles and joints, poor sleep, tension, anxiety, forgetfulness, difficulty in making decisions, aggressiveness, hyperactivity, constantly snacking, craving particular foods, and little desire for sex. Mary found a nutritionist who considered that many symptoms might decrease if she changed her diet. Mary was found to be reacting to several foods: all dairy products, potatoes, tomatoes, tea, peanuts, as well as all pesticides on fruit and vegetables. After four months of avoiding these foods and eating organically produced fruit and vegetables, most of the symptoms had disappeared. Her head and eyes felt clearer than they had for years, her mood swings became a thing of the past, and her crippling backache and other pains vanished. However, she still felt some anxiety. The hot flashes continued, as did the tingling in her legs, and she still felt overweight. Her practitioner then suggested she take a vitamin and mineral test to see how many deficiencies she had. It was discovered that Mary needed magnesium supplements, zinc, selenium, iron, and vitamins C, B1, B2, B3, and B5. Her weight now is rapidly reducing, tingling in her legs does not occur, she is much less anxious, and the hot flashes have almost disappeared. After years of misery, Mary is discovering what it is like to feel well again.

Case study

Philip developed hay fever at the age of two and was not a strong child. Constant infections kept him away from school. At 12 he developed severe depression, migraine symptoms, became very thin, occasionally hallucinated, and eventually was not well enough to go to school at all. Philip was very ill for six years, but he then heard about elimination diets and food rotation. After the first week of eliminating the foods that he was reacting to, he was running about laughing and wanting to study. The headaches stopped, and in the next two weeks all his various medicines were stopped. It took some time to regain good health, but Philip knew he was on the right track and he persisted. He went through a university course, cooking his own food and adhering to the principles of food rotation. He went backpacking across Canada, again carrying the special foods and finding places to cook. He then took some postgraduate courses and settled into a job. Careful maintenance of a rotation diet has made all this possible, as well as homeopathic and radionic treatments. Philip has traveled across America, visited several European countries, and traveled a lot in the United Kingdom. He has not let his diet prevent any of his activities.

problems, they will go away. However, we all know how much easier it is if we nip things in the bud. Take a dandelion growing out of place in a herbaceous border. When it first shows a couple of leaves, it only takes a finger and thumb to remove it; leave it and the roots grow deeper until a garden spade and a surgical operation is needed to remove it, damaging surrounding flowers and plants in the process. We need to take heed of our own early warning signs.

It is now widely accepted that what we eat and how we prepare and cook our food can have an enormous effect on our health. You will have seen how one bite of a sandwich or one sip of a drink can affect your entire body, both physically and mentally. But you also will have seen how to use food to your benefit. The choice is now up to you. Advances in transport and food distribution have brought about an increasing abundance and array of fruits, vegetables, and all kinds of different foods to our stores. So go out and experiment; say good-bye to the foods that can cause you problems—the "convenience" foods full of additives; wheat, corn, and dairy products; the fizzy drinks full of sugar; the chocolate and the potato chips. Instead, let your innate wisdom guide you to the right foods.

Working with the Elimination and Rotation Diets can be a valuable way of getting back to knowing yourself, knowing what your body needs, and gradually becoming more "in tune" with yourself—and therefore with everything else in your life.

Appendix

Foods containing wheat:
wheat flour
wheat bran
wheatmeal
wheat-based crispbreads
wheat biscuits
wheat breakfast cereals (all-bran
    Weetabix, puffed wheat, muesli)
modified starch
baking powder
thickeners and binders
bakery products
some pumpernickel bread
cakes and cake mixes
batter mixes
spaghetti
macaroni and other pasta
pastry
mustard

also check the ingredients of the
following:
baked beans
chocolate and other sweets
cocoa
instant coffee
imitation cream
custard
instant puddings
spreads and pastes
some other flours, e.g., rice flour
bean flours
buckwheat pasta
rye bread
sausages
beef burgers
hamburgers
corned beef
salami
luncheon meat
pâtés

foods coated in breadcrumbs or
    batter
canned soups
sauces—
• oxo cubes
• gravy
• white sauce
• soy sauce
chutneys
alcoholic drinks—
• whiskey
• most gins
• lager
• ale
• beer
• some wines
vitamin and mineral tablets

Foods containing milk and dairy
products:
cow's, goat's, and sheep's milk
condensed, dried, evaporated,
    skimmed, and powdered forms
butter
buttermilk
cream
cheese, including dishes cooked with
    cheese
whey
lactose
casinates
margarines (check whey on labels)
yogurts
custards
cookies
cakes
ice cream
foods cooked in batter
soups
sauces

sausages
prepared meats
most packets of convenience foods
some vitamin and mineral tablets

Note: Homoeopathic remedies can
be obtained in a liquid form free
from sac lac. Doctors can contact
manufacturers to find pain-relieving
medicines that are milk free. Most
tablets contain lactose.

Foods and products containing
corn:
adhesives
envelopes
stamps
stickers
lining of cans for vegetables
lining of paper plates and dishes
toothpaste
talcum powders
laundry starch
aspirin and other tablets
cough syrups
corn flour
sweet corn
popcorn
biscuits
candies
instant coffee and tea
custard
instant puddings
ice cream
cornflakes
ales, beers, whiskey, and some wines
fizzy drinks
batters for frying
corn oil
margarines containing corn oil
peanut butter
salad dressings
bleached white flour
powdered sugar

jam
milk in paper carton
beans and peas from cans
some brands of chips
corn snacks
tortillas
gravy mixes and cubes
sausages
bacon
cured and tenderized ham
creamed soups
stuffing
glucose syrup and glucose in jams
monosodium glutamate
    (Chinese foods)
distilled vinegar
soy sauce
tomato sauce
salt shakers in cafés
pie fillings
fruit juices
canned and frozen fruits
soybean milks
boiled sweets
chewing gum
vitamin C (derived from corn)

Foods containing eggs:
buns
croissants
Danish pastries
biscuits
cakes
flans
pastries and pies
salad dressings
mayonnaise
some prepared salads
custard powder
ice creams
lemon curd
instant whips and processed cream
    preparations
egg white in meringues

macaroons
marshmallows
sorbets
consommé soups
frostings and royal icings
many vaccines are grown on egg
  and may cause reactions
batter mixes made with egg
quiches
fish cakes
egg pasta
enriched alcoholic drinks (eggnogs)

Foods containing yeast:
breads
some biscuits
crispbreads
cakes and cake mixes
flour enriched with vitamins from
  yeast
food coated in bread crumbs
some milk powders are fortified with
  vitamins from yeast (B vitamins)
mushrooms
truffles
cheese of all kinds
buttermilk and cottage cheese
vinegar and all convenience foods
  containing vinegar
gravy browning and similar extracts
yeast/beef extracts
stock cubes
fermented drinks—
• whiskey
• gin
• wine
• brandy
• rum
• vodka
• beer, etc.
malted products—
• cereals
• sweets and chocolates
• milk drinks that have been malted

citrus fruit juice (only home-squeezed
  are yeast free)
many B vitamin products are derived
  from yeast

Foods containing sugar:
most alcoholic drinks
bakery products except stone-ground
  whole-meal bread
instant coffee and tea
hot chocolate
malted milk drinks
milk shakes
soft drinks and low-calorie drinks
fruit juices(except pure fruit juices)
most breakfast cereals
most precooked oven-ready foods
milk products—
• baby milks
• cream
• whipped cream
• ice cream
• processed cheeses
• some fruit yogurts
all desserts
many frozen and packaged foods
many jams
some honey may have sucrose
  added to it
sauces e.g., tomato sauce
soy and other oriental sauces
mayonnaise
relishes
all sweets and candies
all tinned vegetables
fruits
soups
sauces
desserts are likely to contain sugar

about the authors

Jill Carter works as a natural health practitioner in Somerset, England. She is a registered nurse who offers dietary and nutritional counseling; and she also practices healing, therapeutic massage, acupressure, and aromatherapy.

■ ■ ■

Alison Edwards set up the Polden Naturopathic Centre in Somerset, England, more than 20 years ago. She is a registered nurse and a practitioner of complementary medicine, acting as a consultant to clinics throughout Great Britain and overseas.

■ ■ ■ ■ ■ ■

Index

the allergy exclusion diet

■ ■ ■

We hope you enjoyed this Hay House book.
If you would like to receive a free catalog featuring
additional Hay House books and products, or
if you would like information about the
Hay Foundation, please contact:

Hay House, Inc.
P.O. Box 5100
Carlsbad, CA 92018-5100

(760) 431-7695 or (800) 654-5126
(760) 431-6948 (fax) or (800) 650-5115 (fax)
www.hayhouse.com

■ ■ ■

Published and distributed in Australia by: Hay House
Australia Pty Ltd, P.O. Box 515, Brighton-Le-Sands, NSW 2216
phone: 1800 023 516 • *e-mail:* info@hayhouse.com.au

Distributed in Canada by: Raincoast,
9050 Shaughnessy St., Vancouver, B.C., Canada V6P 6E5

■ ■ ■